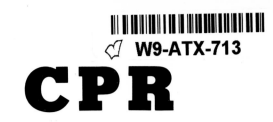

W9-ATX-713

CPR

CPR:

It Could Save Your Life

Donna Armellino, R.N.

Contemporary Books, Inc.
Chicago

Photos by Geoffrey Henderson

Copyright © 1979 by Donna Armellino
All rights reserved
Published by Contemporary Books, Inc.
180 North Michigan Avenue, Chicago, Illinois 60601
Manufactured in the United States of America
Library of Congress Catalog Card Number: 78-74421
International Standard Book Number: 0-8092-7312-8 (cloth)
0-8092-7310-1 (paper)

Published simultaneously in Canada by
Beaverbooks
953 Dillingham Road
Pickering, Ontario L1W 1Z7
Canada

To John, Sr. and his family
so that they can understand it;
and John, Jr., my loving husband,
who encouraged me to write about it.

A special thanks to Gerald and Susan
for modeling in the photographs.

Contents

Introduction

Resuscitation is no longer sacred to the medical and nursing profession—laymen can learn these techniques to save lives. Over 675,000 people die from heart attacks each year. Over half of these deaths occur within the first two hours of the initial onset of pain, usually before the victims are brought to a hospital. Time is the crucial determining factor between life and death.

Cardiac arrest is the sudden cessation of the heart's pumping action. Although cardiac arrest is the end result of all fatal illnesses, too frequently its occurrence is unexpected in people who previously felt healthy and who might otherwise recover. Human lives can be saved by five minutes of simple first aid, but action must be quickly initiated as irreversible brain damage and biological death of body tissue occur within four to six minutes. Heart attack victims can and are successfully resuscitated outside of the hospital; many of them are able to return to a full, productive life.

Resuscitative measures are not limited to heart attack victims, but can be administered in various situations where the heartbeat or breathing has stopped. A few examples of this would be the following: drowning, electric shock, injury from an automobile accident, adverse drug reactions, choking, smoke inhalation, and carbon monoxide poisoning.

The Joint Commission for Accreditation of Hospitals requires nursing personnel and all hospital employees to review and practice resuscitation techniques at least once each year. Through these efforts, off-duty nurses have saved many lives outside the hospital. As concerned citizens, they have revived victims of heart attacks and automobile accidents on interstate highways until paramedic rescue teams have arrived at the scene.

This book is not written in polysyllabic terms aimed at medical, nursing and paramedical health care providers. Basic knowledge of anatomy, normal cardiac activity and factors that influence the heart's function is essential to acquire an understanding of heart disease and has been provided in terms easily understandable by the general public. This information is definitely a prerequisite to actually performing the life-saving C.P.R. measures.

The intent of this book is to teach the basic techniques of cardiopulmonary resuscitation, C.P.R., to interested readers who may have no medical or first-aid training. If more people know how to perform resuscitation before paramedic rescue teams arrive, more lives will be saved. Lay people initiating resuscitation actually save more lives than professional rescue teams with more training, since bystanders can initiate first aid measures immediately. It has been estimated that each year 100,000 lives can be saved nationally through mass public awareness and education in fundamental C.P.R. methods.

Another purpose of this book is to introduce and define the medical terminology used by physicians and nurses in hospital and office settings. The general public is more informed than in the past, but as these concepts become more familiar, people will gain a better understanding of how certain disease processes related to the heart affect the human body. With this increased understanding people can then prepare themselves for discussions with doctors and nurses, asking more intelligent questions of these health care providers, and become more active as participants in their own individualized health care, rather than mere recipients.

Through researching the available literature, we have found many books on the subject of coronary artery disease with related causes, risk factors, and treatment. It is astounding to find that cardio-pulmonary resuscitation has not been included. For this reason, *C.P.R.—It Could Save Your Life* has been written, because it just may help you to save the life of someone you love.

1
History

Man has employed various techniques attempting to resuscitate the dead or near dead for the past four centuries. These rather ingenious methods required common items such as fireside bellows, barrels and
horses. The idea of providing artificial ventilation (forcing air into the lungs — inspiration — and then
manually exerting pressure either indirectly or directly
on the abdomen near the diaphragm to simulate expiration) were established long ago, although not adequately articulated, and still exist today.

Although the basic concepts of artificial ventilation
were established centuries ago, progress was slow in
perfecting the restoration of breathing. In 1530 fireside
bellows were inserted into the victim's mouth and used
to force air into the lungs. The barrel method, a process in which inspiration was produced as chest pressure was released from forward movement of the barrel, was introduced in 1773. Expiration was induced as
body weight compressed the chest with backward
movement. Along European waterways around 1812,
the trotting horse method was used for resuscitation
from near-drownings. The victim was thrown crosswise
over a horse. The weight of the victim's own body
against the horse's back compressed his chest wall
forcing air out. Between the bouncing movements as
the horse trotted, the victim's chest expanded and air
entered his lungs.

In 1861 the *Sylvester method* became quite popular,
and it is still used to a limited extent today. It operates
by utilizing the principle that lung capacity is greater

during inspiration. The victim is lying face-up on a flat, firm surface. The rescuer, while kneeling at his head, alternately raises the victim's arms above his head allowing the chest wall to expand, then lowers the arms, folding them over the chest. Applying pressure indirectly to the chest produces expiration. Several methods followed over the next 50 years, but were merely variations of the above.

Utilizing the principles of positive and negative pressure, a manual device was invented in 1916, then converted into an electrical device in 1926 and operated in an alternating manner, with a vacuum suction causing inspiration and pressure applied directly to the abdomen causing expiration.

In 1959 mouth-to-mouth, or mouth-to-nose, techniques of artificial respiration were developed as the most practical method of providing emergency ventilation without the use of any supportive equipment. Mouth-to-mouth breathing is the simplest and most effective method and has generally replaced the arm lift and back pressure method previously employed.

Then in 1960 a new technique for restoring circulation in someone whose heart had stopped was reported by a team of researchers at the Johns Hopkins Hospital in Baltimore, Maryland. This new technique replaced the old method of opening the chest and massaging the heart directly. Compressing the heart between the breastbone and spinal column proved successful in restoring circulation. The proper combination of external cardiac compression, artificial circulation and mouth-to-mouth breathing, artificial ventilation, was found to sustain a victim of a sudden cardiac arrest for a reasonable period of time. This technique, which has become known as cardio-pulmonary resuscitation — C.P.R.—was endorsed as a medical procedure in 1962 and performed solely by physicians.

But, in 1965 C.P.R. was reclassified as an emergency procedure and the members of emergency care committees recommended that the technique should be applied by properly trained individuals from medical, nursing, dental, allied health professions and rescue squads. This issue was well supported by the American Heart Association, American National Red Cross, Industrial Medical Association, and the U.S. Public Health Service. However, at this time, due to a lack of trained instructors, it was not feasible for the general public to be taught cardio-pulmonary resuscitation techniques.

During the next few years attention was focused on mobile intensive care units, M.I.C.U., so that trained personnel could provide the necessary equipment and emergency care so desperately needed at the scene. When the team reached the patient, he would be treated under the same intensive care conditions as obtained in a hospital coronary care unit. The victim is immediately attached to a portable electrocardiograph monitor that illustrates the electrical activity of the heart and upon which abnormal heartbeats are shown on a screen similar to that of a television. The irregular heartbeats (and the complications that result from them, which may prove fatal) can be detected and controlled through early administration of medications normally stocked in the mobile unit.

If cardiac arrest occurs suddenly, a device capable of producing electric shocks, called a *defibrillator,* is on hand to initiate the heart's pumping action. The mobile unit also provides fast transportation of the victim to a health care facility while the paramedic rescue team members provide continuous, uninterrupted resuscitative measures.

The prototype mobile coronary care unit was initiated in Belfast, Ireland, in 1966. The family doctors in Belfast were acquainted with the facts regarding the risk of unnecessary death immediately after the onset of symptoms suggesting a heart attack. A training scheme in the technique of resuscitation was arranged for medical practitioners, some paramedical workers and appropriate lay individuals. When general practitioners became aware that the majority of coronary deaths were unnecessary and that a mobile unit was available, there was a progressive increase in the number of patients with coronary episodes who came under intensive care soon after the onset of the acute symptoms.

In 1970, Seattle, Washington, public officials started a pilot program of public education. Dr. Leonard A. Cobb, chief of cardiology at Harborview Medical Center and Gordon F. Vickery, the fire chief at that time, headed the program. Firemen took extensive and advanced courses in first aid and cardio-pulmonary resuscitation and were trained to become paramedic technicians. Their rescue measures saved the lives of victims of heart attacks, drowning, electrocution, and many other sudden death emergency situations. Seattle was the first town to enlist people on the street, who witnessed life-threatening emergencies, to perform C.P.R. before a paramedic rescue team arrived.

Within three years, over 18,000 Seattle residents, teenagers and adults, had been taught how to perform C.P.R. Locations selected for instruction included schools, offices, theaters, shopping centers, and private homes. The C.P.R. course is mandatory at some of Seattle's high schools.

That program of public education still exists. Statistics showed that, by August 1976, over 120,000 ordinary Seattle citizens, about one out of every four, had been trained to administer first aid to heart attack and stroke victims. Seattle's goal is to train 200,000 citizens in emergency C.P.R. techniques.

By 1972, in Jacksonville, Florida, more than 150,000 of its 550,000 people had learned C.P.R. methods. Jacksonville is attempting to teach every one of its citizens. The citizen training program was started by Dr. Roy M. Baker to help the half million Jacksonville residents learn how to fight sudden death from cardiac arrest.

Many cardiology experts believe that everyone in America should be knowledgeable in C.P.R. measures. It is particularly important for people in the immediate family of a person who has already survived a heart attack to know these emergency measures. Training sessions for family groups have taken place at club lunches and dinners, sorority meetings, auditoriums, and shopping centers, with television coverage on commercial and educational programs.

In late 1972 the American College of Physicians recommended that a nationwide program be started to educate the general public in C.P.R. Since that time numerous programs have been started across the country, totalling at least 50 cities including Los Angeles, San Francisco, Houston, Miami, Grand Rapids, Newark, and Columbus to cite a few. In the rapidly expanding field of health care the responsibility really belongs to the community itself. If someone suffers a serious heart attack, the best chance for survival rests with educated bystanders.

Firemen resuscitate more people than doctors, because they get to the scene of many medical emergencies sooner. But even firemen cannot reach every clinically dead victim within minutes. This could be one of the factors attributing to the high mortality rate accounting for over 50 percent of deaths before the victims arrive at a hospital. Timeliness in starting C.P.R. is indispensable. A brain-damaged person, at best, is the result if there is no one at the scene who has been trained in C.P.R. The mortality rate will substantially decrease as more people are educated in the techniques of performing C.P.R. Better emergency care at the scene will reduce the nation's coronary mortality rate. If C.P.R. is started within one minute of cardiac arrest there is a 98 percent chance of full recovery. If nothing is done for a person whose heart has stopped beating, or lungs have stopped breathing, death is inevitable.

The National Conference on Cardio-Pulmonary Resuscitation and Emergency Cardiac Care established standards for C.P.R. in 1974. These standards are rules of safety that apply universally to all emergency situations. A copy of these standards may be obtained from the local chapters of the American Heart Association, a list of which has been included at the back of this book.

The Y.M.C.A. is currently launching a nationwide C.P.R. training program. Workers of electric-utility, city water and sewer departments are learning the techniques of C.P.R. Ski patrolmen, insurance companies, scouts, airline stewardesses and other flight personnel are being taught resuscitative measures in their first aid courses. It is also required knowledge of many owners and their employees in local grocery stores.

The general public is becoming more aware of the use of C.P.R. and its success. The benefits of modern resuscitation methods can readily be seen on television's *Emergency One* series with the paramedics in action. In early 1977, the CBS Television Network devoted its *60 Minutes* program to C.P.R. And in September, 1977, a certified instructor from the American National Red Cross demonstrated the technique on the *Dinah!* Show.

Volunteers having varied backgrounds donate their time for the American National Red Cross to instruct the public in cardio-pulmonary resuscitation. In many areas at the present time, a formal schedule of dates for class sessions does not exist due to a shortage of trained instructors. However, interested persons should contact their local chapters of the American National Red Cross. These centers are listed in the telephone directory. Receptionists for the Red Cross will contact students with information on when the sessions are scheduled. The sessions consist of twelve hours in total; meetings are held for a single three-hour session per week for four consecutive weeks. In the fiscal year ending July 30, 1977, 123 teaching sessions were completed by the Mid-America Chapter which covers four of the larger counties in Illinois. In those sessions, 12,098 people were certified to perform C.P.R. techniques.

In the March 5, 1978, edition of the Chicago *Sun-Times' Parade* Magazine, editor Jess Gorkin advocated formal high school instruction in C.P.R. techniques. He felt that the life-saving measures should be incorporated into the health and physical education curriculum and that it should be mandatory for graduation in all private and public high schools.

The goal of the American Heart Association is to teach C.P.R. to one out of every two persons by 1985. The massive effort would seem to be worthwhile. The facts resulting from the Seattle training program show that over 200 people have been successfully resuscitated, at a rate of two persons each week during a two-year period. A nationwide program to promote mass public awareness and education will probably save 100,000 lives a year in the U.S.

2
The Cardio-Vascular System

Function

The heart is the most efficient pump known to man. It functions as a continuous pump for the circulatory system propelling blood through the blood vessels of the body. From the fourth week of embryonic development, the heart is formed and pulsations have begun, and it pumps endlessly until death without rest. Even the world's most expensive and best run automobile must be taken into the repair shop for a periodic tune-up.

Each of the two upper chambers, *atrium,* receive the blood that is returned to the heart. They are small chambers with thin walls. The lower chambers, the ventricles, are larger chambers with thick walls that send the blood to various parts of the body. The capacity of each chamber is about two ounces.

The heart pumps about 70-90 times per minute, or about 100,000 times each day. Slightly over seven tons of blood is moved each day through the circulatory system, amounting to 2600 tons of blood each year.

Blood is distributed to body tissues by the *arteries* whose elastic, muscular walls expand and contract, causing increases and decreases in blood pressure. Blood is returned to the heart through a similar structure of *veins.*

The chief function of the blood is to deposit carbon dioxide and pick up oxygen in the lungs and carry it to the cells in various parts of the body to meet the metabolic demands for survival.

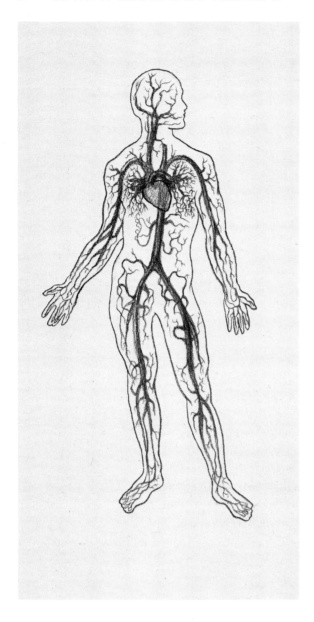

THE CIRCULATORY SYSTEM

Location

The heart lies directly underneath the breastbone, or *sternum,* and on top of the backbone, or *spinal column.* It lies slightly off-center, with one-third of its mass to the right and the remaining two-thirds to the left of the middle of the chest. Centered between the right and left lungs, the heart is surrounded in the upper chest, or *thorax,* by the rib cage and muscles. Its lowermost border is pointed toward the left side of the body at the level of the fifth rib, and rests on the diaphragm. The heart is rotated toward the left side, making it lie slightly on its right side.

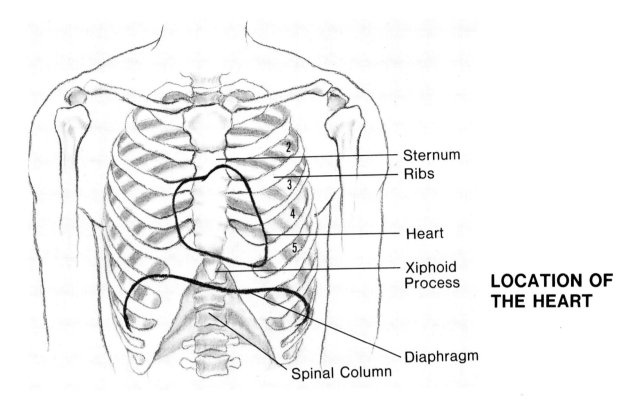

Sternum
Ribs
Heart
Xiphoid Process
Diaphragm
Spinal Column

LOCATION OF THE HEART

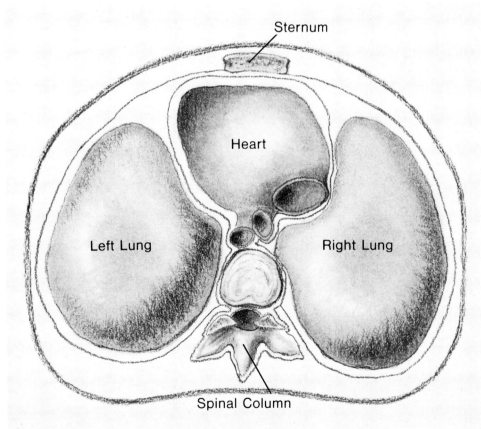

Sternum
Heart
Left Lung
Right Lung
Spinal Column

CROSS-SECTIONAL VIEW OF LOCATION OF THE HEART

In the adult, the length of the heart measures five inches with a three and one-half inch breadth and a two and one-half inch thickness. The heart weighs approximately three quarters of a pound and its size is about the same as a tightly clenched fist. The rounded top portion forms the base and the somewhat pointed lower portion forms the apex, resembling the shape of a cone. The precise dimensions and shape vary from one individual to another based on his or her own height, weight, and body build.

In persons with broad chests, the heart lies on a more horizontal plane. Persons with long, narrow chests have long, narrow hearts which lie more vertically in the body and do not extend as far into the left side of the thoracic cage.

Structure

Surrounding the entire structure of the heart is the *pericardial sac.* It is a protective fluid-filled cover and facil-

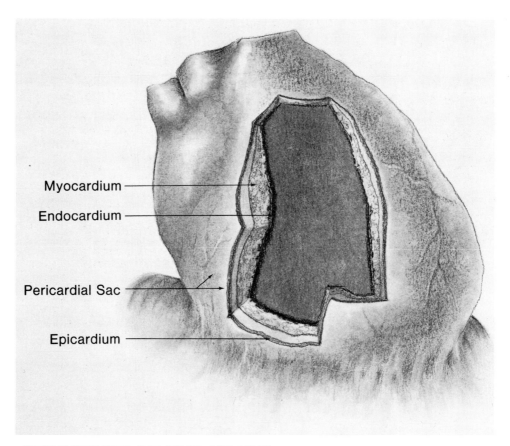

Myocardium

Endocardium

Pericardial Sac

Epicardium

STRUCTURE OF THE HEART

itates the movements of the heart as it contracts and relaxes. This sac acts as a cushion reducing friction that would result from the pumping action. The pericardial sac functions in the same manner as shock absorbers in an automobile that help to minimize the bumps of the road.

The heart is made up of three layers of cells: *epicardium, myocardium,* and *endocardium.* The epicardium is the thin outermost layer. The middle layer, myocardium, is composed of thick muscle tissue and is responsible for actually causing the heart to forcefully pump the blood out into the circulatory system. Since the contractions must be more forceful from the ventricles, the myocardium in the ventricular walls is much thicker than in the atria. Because the blood must travel from the left ventricle throughout the entire circulatory system, the myocardium is thickest in the wall of the left ventricle. The endocardium is a thin, smooth, moist, reddish membrane lining the internal surface of the heart. It is thickest in the atria and is actually bathed by the blood.

The circulatory system can be considered a closed system surrounding the heart and consists of approximately 72,000 miles of blood vessels. All blood leaves the heart by arteries and returns to the heart by veins. The blood travels from the heart via the *aorta,* the largest artery in the body. Approximately the size of a large garden hose, the diameter is about one to two inches and somewhat resembles the trunk of a tree as it branches off into smaller segments. These segments, *arterioles,* carry the blood to the tissues.

A twig-like maze of microscopic cells make up the bed of *capillaries* separating the *arterial blood system* (oxygenated blood carried away from the heart through the arteries) from the *venous blood system* (oxygen-deficient blood transported toward the heart through veins). It is here, in the capillary bed, that the exchange takes place. Oxygen and nourishment are given to the tissues and carbon dioxide and waste products are removed. As the blood leaves the capillary bed it enters venules, then larger segments, the veins, as the blood is returned to the heart for replenishment.

The structure of the artery is tubular in shape, with an extremely smooth lining to reduce friction. The internal diameter of the artery is called the *lumen* and adjusts to the amount of blood flowing through it. The

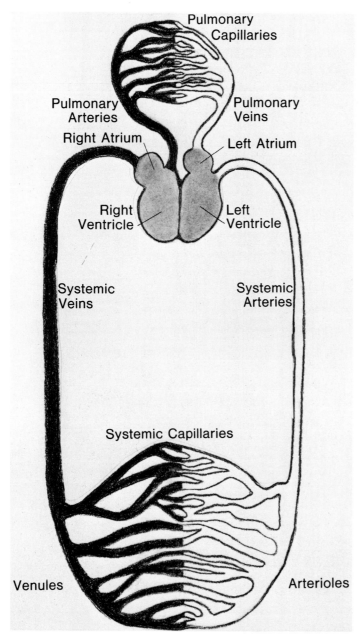

CIRCULATION OF THE BLOOD

wall of an artery consists of three layers: *intima, media* and *adventia.* The inner layer, intima, is composed of an elastic membrane. The middle layer, media, is composed of elastic tissue fibers and smooth muscle cells. The outermost layer is the adventia and is composed of loose connective tissue. The size of the diameter of the vessel changes by contraction and relaxation of the smooth muscle in its walls. Comparatively, the arteries are larger in size than the veins, facilitating a larger surface area with less resistance allowing the blood to flow easily.

BLOOD VESSELS

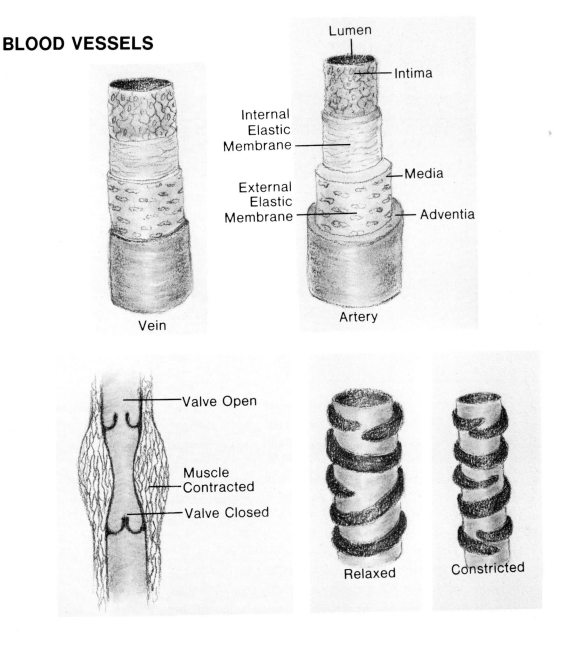

Vein

Artery

Valve Open

Muscle Contracted

Valve Closed

Relaxed

Constricted

Like its counterpart, the vein is also tubular in shape. All blood is returned to the heart by veins, which have valves which prohibit the backward motion of blood. These valves are essential, since the blood in the lower extremities must be returned against the force of gravity.

Components

The heart serves as a pump to deliver blood to the body tissues in an attempt to meet their metabolic de-

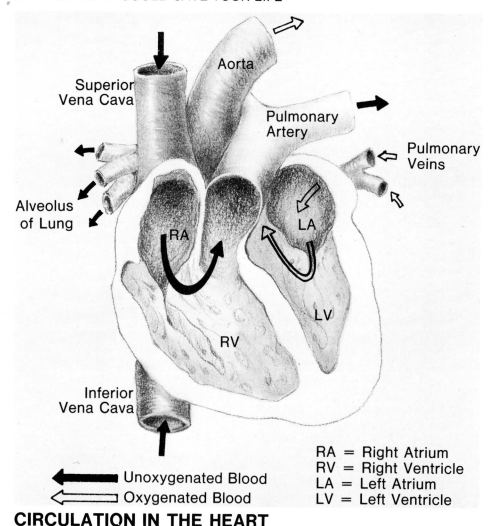

RA = Right Atrium
RV = Right Ventricle
LA = Left Atrium
LV = Left Ventricle

Unoxygenated Blood
Oxygenated Blood

CIRCULATION IN THE HEART

mands. The heart is a hollow structure with a wall, the septum, dividing it into two sides, right and left. As previously mentioned, each side consists of two chambers, the upper, atrium, and the lower, the ventricles. The right and left sides of the heart differ in both function and muscular structure.

Blood carrying carbon dioxide and waste products from tissue and cell metabolism is returned to the heart by veins. This venous, or oxygen-deficient blood, is transported from the body by two large veins. The *superior vena cava* returns blood from the brain and upper extremities. The *inferior vena cava* transports blood from the abdominal organs and lower extremities. Both large veins empty their contents into the right atrium. The venous blood flows from the atrium into the ventricle and is then pumped out into the *pulmonary system* (primarily the lungs) via the *pulmonary arteries.* Therefore the function of the right side of the heart is to deliver the unoxygenated, venous blood to the lungs.

In the lungs the blood deposits carbon dioxide and waste products accumulated from tissue and cell metabolism. In exchange it picks up oxygen, giving it the red color. The oxygenated blood is now returned to the heart by one of four *pulmonary veins.* The pulmonary veins empty into the left atrium. The arterial blood flows from the atrium into the ventricle and is then forcefully pumped out into the circulatory system via the aorta to deliver oxygen to cells and vital organs. Therefore, the function of the left side of the heart is to deliver oxygenated blood from the lungs to the body.

But since the blood must flow through the entire arterial system, the force of the contraction of the left ventricle must be strong enough to propel its contents the entire distance. The heart has to work against great pressure and resistance, therefore, the muscular structure of the wall of the left ventricle must be thick and strong to force the oxygenated blood to the body. In comparison, since the distance is shorter and the pressure in the pulmonary system is minimal, the muscular wall of the right ventricle is considerably thinner.

Cardiac Activity

There are two types of activity taking place simultaneously in the heart, electrical and mechanical. Just as a car's electrical system triggers the mechanical movement of the engine, electrical activity in the heart dictates its mechanical pumping action. The normal healthy heart works in a fundamental, rhythmical pattern.

Nerve cells are specialized fibers that proceed along pathways to and from the brain through all parts of the body. Nerves carrying impulses toward the nerve centers are called *afferent;* nerves carrying impulses away from nerve centers are called *efferent.* The function of the nerve is two-fold: to convey sensation and to originate motion. For example, after touching a hot burner on a stove, it would seem like a reflex action to pull the hand away from the burner. A split second passes by, but in that time the heat sensors in the fingertips actually send a message to the brain telling it the surface is hot. The brain then signals the muscles in the arm and hand to pull away from the source of heat.

Muscle cells in the heart differ from muscle cells elsewhere in the body. The latter are dependent on nerve impulses originating in the brain. But the myocardial cells are capable of initiating contraction without any outside nervous stimulation. This concept of independent muscular contractions is called *automaticity.* However, the heart rate is influenced by the nervous sytem in response to other needs of the body.

The heart has an intrinsic electrical system that allows for an impulse to originate in the right atrium at the junction, or *sinus,* of the superior and inferior vena cava. This group of cells is referred to as the *sino-atrial,* or *S.A., node.* It is a specialized network of nerve cells and functions as the pacemaker of the heart regulating its rhythmical contractions. The S.A. node, without any outside influence, will discharge impulses at a rate of 70-80 times per minute. Each impulse is then transmitted over both atria, similar to the ripples formed when a pebble is thrown into a pond. The impulse then activates another network of nerve cells called the *atrio-ventricular,* or *A.V., node.* This second impulse is then transmitted in the same fashion over both ventricles. The impulses travel from the A.V. node towards the wall separating the ventricles. After reaching the septum, it travels along both sides of the septum to the *perkinje fibers.* These fibers connect the upper and lower segments of the ventricles. As the impulse travels from the perkinje fibers, the walls of the ventricle are stimulated. This stimulation of the nerve pathways results in muscular contraction.

Up until this time the heart has been discussed in terms of the right and left sides. Since the right and left sides of the heart work together at the same time, now it is necessary to discuss the heart in terms of upper and lower halves.

The muscles respond to the nerve stimulation and the result is the mechanical pumping activity. This pumping action consists of two phases: a period of contraction, *systole,* and a period of relaxation, *diastole.* Contraction is the shortening of the length of a muscle. For example, as a rubberband is stretched, the fibers become longer and thinner. It reaches a point where it cannot expand any further. Unless it breaks, it suddenly snaps resuming its original shape. This exam-

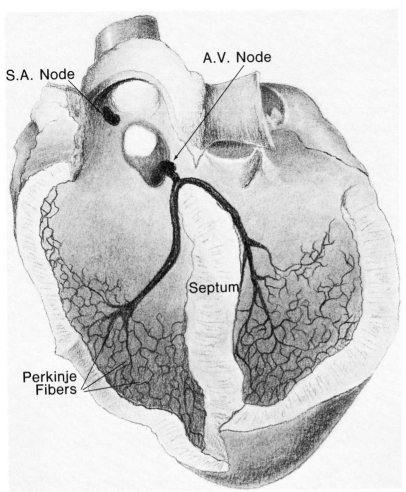

S.A. Node

A.V. Node

Septum

Perkinje
Fibers

ELECTRICAL SYSTEM

ple illustrates the expansion and contraction of the muscular walls of the chambers of the heart.

The pumping activity of the heart is a timed sequence of events, systole and diastole, and is coordinated with both atria filling and contracting together at the same time, as well as the ventricles working simultaneously. As the atria contract, the ventricles fill, and as the ventricles contract, the atria fill. As the blood from the superior and inferior vena cava empties into the right atrium the walls of the atrium expand allowing the size of this chamber to enlarge to accommodate the volume of blood. Atrial filling is referred to as *atrial diastole.* When the atrium can no longer expand, it contracts, forcing all of its contents into the lower chamber, the ventricle.

This squeezing action by the atria as it empties its contents is referred to as *atrial systole* (emptying). Simultaneously, the ventricles begin to fill, the walls ex-

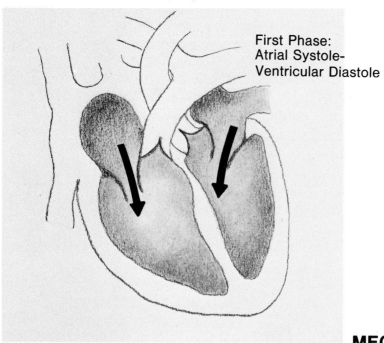

First Phase:
Atrial Systole-
Ventricular Diastole

MECHANICAL PUMPING ACTION

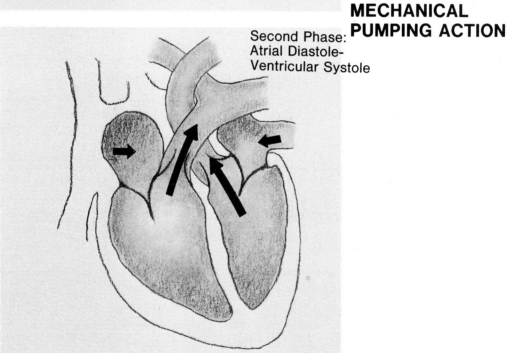

Second Phase:
Atrial Diastole-
Ventricular Systole

pand, and the chamber enlarges. Ventricular filling is known as *ventricular diastole.* Together these two components make up the first phase — atrial systole and ventricular diastole.

Ventricular systole takes place after the chambers expand to their fullest capacity and the muscular walls contract. This contraction makes the chamber smaller, thus forcing its contents simultaneously into the circulatory system and pulmonary system. During ventricular systole the atria are filling. Together these two components make up the second phase — ventricular systole and atrial diastole. This process is repeated incessantly so long as life persists. The filling and emptying of a meat baster as the bulb is squeezed will make this difficult concept easier to understand.

Electrical activity can be recorded by an instrument called an *electrocardiograph.* Disposable electrodes are attached to the chest wall. These circular discs are made of extremely sensitive material capable of detecting minute electrical impulses. These impulses are then amplified and recorded by a needle in the electrocardiograph as lines or deflections on a continuously moving roll of graph paper. This strip of paper is a graphic representation of the electrical activity of the heart and is called an *electrocardiogram, E.C.G.,* or *E.K.G.*

The E.C.G. records the transmission of electrical impulses along the nerve pathways. It illustrates the impulse originating at the S.A. node traveling across the atria causing systole, to the A.V. node and through the ventricles causing ventricular systole, then diastole. The E.C.G. indicates the heart rate which is defined as the number of heartbeats occurring in a given period of time, usually one minute. The regularity of the heartbeat is referred to as the rhythm. Atrial and ventricular rhythm are each considered separately and are determined as regular or irregular by counting the number of spaces between the heartbeats on the graphic sheet.

Electrical abnormalities can be detected by examining the E.C.G. strip. Impulses originating at a site other than the S.A. node, or a delay in transmission of the impulse as it travels down the nerve pathways will be quite evident to a person experienced in reading electrocardiograms. Sometimes an irregular heartbeat can be felt in the chest and is experienced as a "skipped beat" or "fluttering sensation." The medical term for an irregular heartbeat is a *palpitation.* Palpitations are usually felt while the body is at rest such as sitting in a chair reading a newspaper, and subside with activity such as walking. These irregularities are not usually indications of heart disease, but if they are persistent, the condition should be investigated by a physician and an E.C.G. taken.

In the undamaged heart the ventricles respond to the stimulus provided by the A.V. node which is dependent on the S.A. node. But in the damaged heart, the atria and ventricles sometimes work independently. The conduction system that transmits the nerve stimuli to keep the heart beating in a rhythmical pattern suddenly loses control — although there is nothing physi-

LARGE ARTERIES

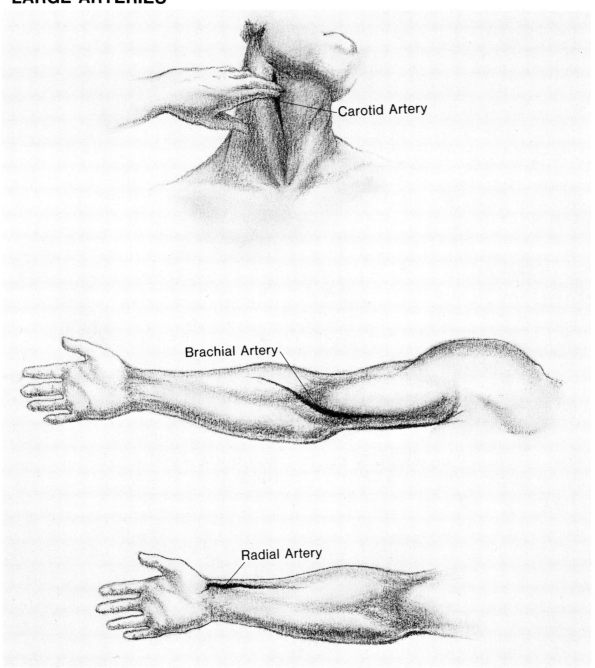

cally wrong with the heart muscle itself. The heart merely stops — similar to a stereo system that has been short-circuited. If restarted in time, the heart can again continue to function indefinitely.

Pulse

A throbbing-like pulsation can be felt over the larger arteries, and is called the pulse. The pulse is actually the expansion and contraction of the arterial walls that correspond with the heartbeat. It is a result of ventricular systole, the strong contraction propelling the blood into the circulatory system delivering blood to the brain and vital organs to sustain life.

The aorta is the largest artery in the body, stemming directly from the left ventricle of the heart. Its primary function is to carry blood to the abdominal organs such as the liver, spleen, and kidneys. Almost immediately, as it departs from the heart, smaller arteries branch off from it. These branches lie closer to the body's skin surface and can be found and felt without too much difficulty.

Supplying the brain, the *carotid artery* can be located on the neck approximately one to one and one-half inches to either side of the Adam's apple. In an emergency situation the carotid pulse is most frequently measured because of its obvious exposure and the fact that it is not usually covered by clothing. The *brachial artery* delivers blood to the arms and can be found on the inner aspect of the bend of the elbow, the inner one-third of the arm closest to the body. Carrying blood to the hands, the *radial artery* is smaller, but with some practice can be felt easily. It is located at the inner aspect of the wrist closest to the thumb. This is the site usually selected by doctors and nurses while counting a person's pulse. In the groin, the *femoral artery* delivers blood to the legs and feet. Its size is large, but usually covered by clothing, making it more difficult to feel.

The above listed arteries are the largest in the body and can be felt without much difficulty. To feel a pulse, the index and middle fingers are placed gently, but firmly, across the artery. If present, a slight tapping sensation will be felt against the fingertips. If too great a pressure is applied, the circulation will be blocked and the pulse will not be detected. Taking a pulse is not technically difficult, but does require a certain amount of practice.

Blood Pressure

As the blood is pumped out of the heart it is forced into the vessels. The blood under pressure from the heart pushes against the walls of the vessels. Blood pressure is the measurement of how hard the blood pushes against the vessel walls. Many factors influence blood pressure, such as obesity, smoking, diet, stress, and certain disease processes which can cause it to become elevated. Low blood pressure occurs when the heart action is weak or the arterioles are dilated during a fever, or shock. The blood pressure normally fluctuates slightly during daily activities. Exercise and excitement tend to raise blood pressure temporarily. It is usually lowest in the morning after a good night's rest and is highest during the early evening hours.

Three chief forces serve to maintain the blood pressure:

1. the strength of the contraction of the heart muscle;

2. the elasticity of the arterial walls;

3. the peripheral resistance that exists due to the smaller diameter of the arterioles as the blood travels from the arteries.

An inflatable cuff is used to measure the pressure. The Greek word *sphygmomanometer* has been given to name this instrument and means "to measure the thin pulse." The inflatable cuff is applied snugly around the upper part of the arm, approximately one inch above the inner aspect at the bend of the elbow, the *antecubital space.* This is the site of the brachial artery. The arm must be kept straight and at rest for at least one minute as muscle movement will cause pressure around the arteries eliciting a slight elevation.

When the cuff is inflated the blood supply to the lower arm and hand is blocked and no pulse can be felt either at the brachial or radial arteries. A tight, constricting feeling will be experienced similar to when a tourniquet is applied to obtain a specimen of blood. If left in place too long, a tingling sensation will occur, indicating that the circulation to the hand is not sufficient. Pressure should be released from the inflated cuff for a few minutes, then attempts to measure the blood pressure repeated. The cuff is then slowly deflated until the pulse can be felt or the blood rushing through the vessel can be heard by the use of a stethoscope. A column of mercury or an aeroid manometer is attached to the sphygmomanometer to determine the two numbers indicating the blood pressure measurement.

The first number is referred to as the *systolic pressure.* As its name implies, it is the highest pressure along the vessel walls as the heart contracts, the period during which the ventricles expel their contents into the aorta and the pulmonary artery.

The second number indicates the *diastolic pressure* as the ventricles of the heart fill between contractions. Without constriction of the artery, this is the lowest pressure along the vessel walls as normal blood flow is resumed. This second reading corresponds with the phase of relaxation in the heartbeat—the brief interval in which the heart relaxes and rests between its contractions.

Normal blood pressure in a healthy young adult is 120 millimeters of mercury systolic pressure and 80 millimeters of mercury diastolic pressure, and is read merely as 120 over 80. The upper limits of normal for adults is generally considered 140/90. Blood pressure measurements that remain persistently elevated above 150/90, either systolic or diastolic, need to be brought to the attention of the family physician.

High blood pressure is called *hypertension.* It does not mean that the person is extremely nervous or high strung. At least three separate yet consecutively elevated readings at five to seven day intervals are necessary to interpret the measurements as hypertensive. Several community fire and health care departments have established free weekly sessions to check blood pressures. The readings may be recorded and brought to the doctor's office on the next visit.

Over 23 million Americans have high blood pressure. Over half of these people do not know it and only one-half of the people who do know it follow their prescribed treatment plan. If untreated, high blood pressure will affect the heart, kidneys, or possibly cause a stroke. The basic pathology of high blood pressure is the narrowing of the small arteries that increases the pressure in them and makes it more difficult for the heart to pump blood through them.

The specific cause of high blood pressure in 90-95 percent of the people that have it is unknown. It is considered a silent disease and even a silent killer, as usually there are no symptoms experienced. If present, symptoms consist of headaches, usually located at the back of the head, and are generally more severe upon rising in the morning, and then disappear a few hours later. Other symptoms that may occur are occasional dizziness (vertigo), nosebleeds, spots before the eyes, or a feeling of tension. If symptoms are present, they do not indicate how high the blood pressure measures.

High blood pressure cannot be cured, but it can be controlled with close medical supervision and following the physician's prescribed treatment plan. This plan may include a calorie-controlled weight reduction diet, limited salt intake, a regular daily exercise program, and/or medications. Stress is also an influencing factor on blood pressure, and attempts should be made to reduce it and keep it at a minimum. Cigarette smoking should be stopped, as the nicotine causes the arteries to constrict.

With age, the arteries lose their elasticity, peripheral resistance tends to become greater and the heart muscle has to pump with greater force to circulate blood through the body. As a consequence, the blood pressure gradually rises. Blood pressure measurements should be checked regularly, as ordered by the doctor.

Heart Circulation

The heart itself must receive oxygenated blood for its own maintenance. The coronary vessels are the first branches off the aorta as it departs from the heart. The term *coronary* literally means crown, and the coronary arteries actually encircle the heart to supply it with oxygen and nutrients. The heart's blood supply provides blood for both its electrical conduction and mechanical contraction activities. The heart's circulatory system is independent from the rest of the body's circulation. Therefore, a steady and adequate supply must be maintained. If the blood supply to the heart is blocked, cardiac cells die, contraction ceases, and the entire circulation comes to a standstill.

There are two main coronary arteries, right and left, each having small segments, anterior, the front, and posterior, the back. The downward portion of the seg-

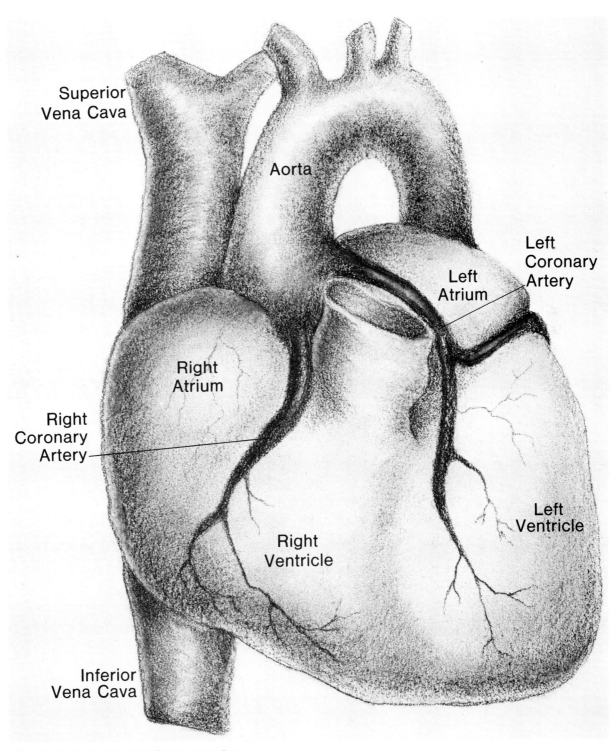

CORONARY CIRCULATION

ments is called descending. The coronary arteries approximate the diameter of a drinking straw. Blood flow through these narrow arteries is estimated at approximately one cup per minute, with only 15 percent traveling through the right artery and the remaining 85 percent traveling through the left artery.

The term *occlusion* means to close. The vessels may become closed by spasm of the vessel wall or by a blood clot. Closure of the coronary vessels can, and often does, prove fatal. Coronary occlusion results in a dead area of the heart, an *infarction,* which weakens the contraction of the heart muscle and less blood is pumped when the body is at rest. But during exercise, more oxygen is required, thus placing more of a demand on the heart to meet the body's requirements.

Blood flow can be greatly reduced by *atherosclerosis,* a process whereby the inner walls of the blood vessels become thickened and lose their elastic quality, which causes the internal diameter of the vessels to become even narrower. Deposits of fats, fibers, and calcium collect along the inner lining of the coronary arteries to form plaques. This is a gradual process that occurs over many years and will go unnoticed until the arteries become severely narrowed. This can, and often does, lead to formation of a blood clot, a *thrombosis.* Subsequent blood supply to the heart muscle beyond this blockage is impaired, and the result is severe damage or death of the heart muscle, infarction. The area normally supplied by the artery, prior to its blockage, does not regenerate, and the dead tissue becomes a burden to the heart.

Then, symptoms will develop which provide warning that the heart muscle is not getting enough oxygen. One clinical syndrome that results from a relatively inadequate blood supply to the heart is known as *angina pectoris,* characterized by a sudden attack of pain located at the sternum. Usually described as pressure or tightness, the pain may travel or radiate to either the right or left arm or neck. This pain is triggered by physical exertion, overeating, stress, or other emotional factors where the heart rate increases causing a greater demand for oxygen. Anginal pain is usually of short duration, lasting five to ten minutes and usually rapidly relieved by rest or administration of nitroglycerin, a medication that opens the coronary arteries.

If continuously ignored, or passed off as gastric indigestion, severe damage to the heart muscle will result, leading to actual death of the muscle cells. Angina pectoris often precedes a complete coronary occlusion and is referred to as pre-infarction pain. This process is referred to as *myocardial infarction,* more commonly known as a heart attack. Acute myocardial infarction is a clinical syndrome characterized by pain, which is not usually associated with exertion and frequently occurs during sleep. The pain experienced with a heart attack is sudden and severe in nature and has been described as crushing or vise-like. The intense pain is usually felt underneath the sternum, but may radiate to either the right or left arm or the jaw or back just as anginal pain, but the severity is much more intense.

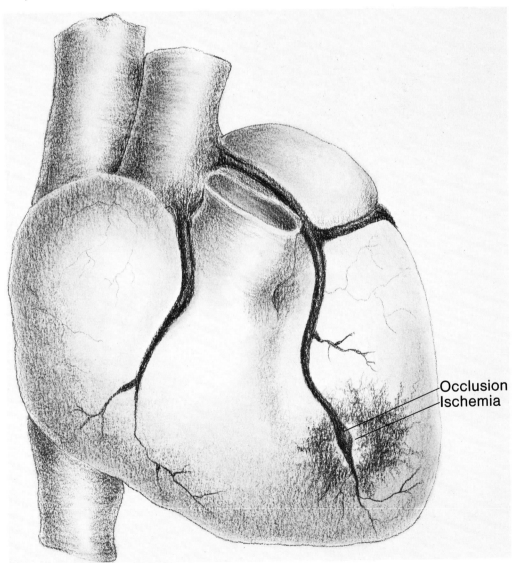

Occlusion
Ischemia

MYOCARDIAL INFARCTION

Other symptoms accompanying the pain include nausea, vomiting, weakness, anxiety, profuse sweating, and difficulty in breathing.

Myocardial infarction is the death, or *necrosis,* of the cardiac muscle resulting from an interrupted or diminished supply of oxygenated blood. Usually occurring as a result of a pathologic condition in the coronary artery system, the majority of cases of acute heart attack, due to coronary blockage, stem from arteriosclerotic heart disease. Since the left ventricle is responsible for performing most of the heart's work, cardiac problems are usually located there. In fact, heart attacks occur almost exclusively in the left ventricle. The extent of the muscle damage depends on the site of the occlusion in the coronary artery. If the main branch is blocked, all subsequent blood flow is obstructed and the infarcted area will be quite extensive. If the blockage is in a smaller segment the infarcted area will be considerably less.

The heart has a compensatory mechanism whereby the force of the blood pushing against the blockage places pressure along the sides of the vessel walls. This pressure aids in establishing new, smaller branches of the coronary arteries that form interconnected pathways. Similar to that of a spider's web, this collateral circulation is established, but it takes a long time for these new routes to perform the same function of delivering the same amount of blood to the heart muscles.

Risk Factors

A risk factor is something that causes a person to have a higher probability of contracting a disease. Just as black people are more prone to have high blood pressure, the white male is more likely to have a heart attack. Some of these risk factors cannot be remedied, others can be controlled through a change in lifestyle, daily habits, and close medical supervision.

Our life span has lengthened to an average of 73 years. Through better education, public health measures and sustained standards of living, the life span will lengthen even further.

A complete, yearly physical examination should be obtained, including laboratory tests of blood sugar and cholesterol levels, along with an electrocardiogram.

Even with the rising cost of medical services (along with everything else), the cost of a physical checkup is a minimal price to pay considering the alternative cost of hospitalization, or with complete ignorance and negligence, death.

There are certain factors in one's life that cannot be changed. At conception the body hormones determine the sex as either male or female. The risk of coronary artery disease is much higher in males, particularly in the 50-60 year age group. But studies have shown that by age 15 coronary artery disease is usually present. In fact, over 40 percent of deaths among American males twenty years of age or older result from coronary artery disease. Estrogen, a female hormone, helps protect the coronary arteries against the formation of fat deposits in women before menopause. Within seven to ten years after the change of life, the protective effect of estrogen decreases until the percentage of coronary artery disease present is similar to males in the same age group.

There are other personal factors that cannot be altered. A person is powerless to change his or her race or family history. The incidence of heart disease is much higher in Caucasians than in any other race. Certain disease processes seem to have some genetic bearing. Researchers have linked certain disorders to heredity such as diabetes, epileptic seizures, kidney and heart disease. If either grandparent has such an illness, it may be passed down to his or her sons or daughters, and to their offspring as well.

Offspring usually follow the examples that are set for them. Children of short, grossly overweight parents usually do not develop into tall, slender adults. Body build plays an important role in health maintenance. *Mesomorph* is a term used to describe the structural framework of a person who is of short stature with large thick bones. He is usually overweight and has a sedentary existence, a lack of regular daily exercise. This contributes to the development of coronary artery disease. Obesity is defined as an increase of ten to twenty percent over ideal body weight. Excess weight causes an increase in blood cholesterol levels and elevated blood pressure. Obesity throws an even greater workload on a heart which has to pump blood through narrow, hardened arteries to meet the body's demands. Exercise is essential to keep the body in a healthy state. It helps to lower blood cholesterol and blood pressure, control weight, and relieve stress and tension. Regular, daily exercise such as walking, jogging, or swimming reduces the chance of having a heart attack by two-thirds.

Cholesterol, a fatty alcohol, is produced by the liver only in the amount necessary to meet body requirements. Excess amounts of cholesterol come from ingestion of saturated fats found in meat, whole milk and whole milk products. Although it is essential in making digestive acids and hormones, an excess tends to raise the cholesterol level in the blood. If too great a quantity is present, it collects along the inner walls of the arteries and leads to arteriosclerosis, hardening and narrowing of the arteries which results in a reduced blood flow. Such a condition can also lead to the formation of a clot which may block or occlude an already restricted artery and may cause a heart attack or a stroke. Because of the hormone estrogen, produced by women during the child bearing years, women usually are not as vulnerable to develop arteriosclerosis until they have passed menopause. To reduce the amount of cholesterol consumed by eating, one should change his dietary habits to include 2 percent lowfat milk or skim milk, margarine, poultry and fish, with only three animal meat servings per week. And of course, the number of eggs should be limited also, to three per week.

Diabetes is a disease process whereby the pancreas does not secrete an adequate amount of insulin to meet the body's requirements. People inflicted with this disorder need to develop an understanding of how the disease alters their body metabolism to avoid complications. Through altering their dietary habits, maintaining regular daily exercise and close medical supervision, they can control the disease. But like many diseases, diabetes is a long process and can affect other parts of the body. In diabetes, the arteries eventually become hardened and lose their elastic quality. The combination of diabetes and an elevated cholesterol level, causes the arteries to become damaged even more rapidly.

Cigarette smoking increases the risk of developing coronary artery disease by affecting the lungs' ability to exchange air. Nicotine, the toxic substance of cigarette smoke, makes the heart beat faster and causes certain arteries, such as coronary arteries, to become narrow. Narrowing of the arteries causes the blood pressure to become elevated, putting more work load on the heart muscle. The death rate from coronary artery disease is three times higher in cigarette smokers than nonsmokers. Cigar and pipe smokers do not have a higher death rate from coronary artery disease.

High blood pressure, hypertension, increases the rate at which arteriosclerosis develops in coronary arteries. Normal blood pressure in a healthy young adult is 120/80. A blood pressure that remains persistently elevated above 150/90 (either systolic or diastolic) results from increased resistance in the periphery of the circulatory system.

The incidence of heart attacks is three times higher in people with hypertension than it is in people with normal blood pressure. Hypertension can be controlled with close medical supervision and following the physician's prescribed treatment plan, which may include a weight reducing diet, limited salt intake, regular daily exercise, and/or medications. Since there is no cure for high blood pressure at the present time, treatment is directed toward lowering the blood pressure, and if present, minimizing symptoms that have developed from it. Unfortunately, as the medications eliminate the annoying symptoms of headaches and dizziness the person begins to feel better and decides he no longer needs to take the medication. This false reasoning is often exhibited by hypertensive patients, and, therefore, it cannot be stressed enough that medications must be taken as prescribed by the physician. If uncomfortable side effects are experienced, the physician should be notified. The doctor may then decide to alter the medication dosage or change to another type of anti-hypertensive drug.

Few people relish the idea of taking pills. Sometimes medication is the only answer to lowering the blood pressure to a safe level. The purpose of taking the drug is to prevent the development of coronary artery disease in addition to other complications directly related to hypertension and assist the individual to live a longer, healthier life.

Personality and behavioral coping mechanisms also play key factors in the development of coronary artery disease. Recently, a great deal of research has been conducted correlating personality types with the development of angina and myocardial infarctions. Several risk categories have been established. Type A individuals possess character traits of aggressiveness and competitiveness, and will often actively seek promotions and feel compelled to meet exacting deadlines. Type B individuals are relaxed, easy-going, satisfied people who are not compelled to work within a strict schedule. Studies completed over the past few years have concluded that there is twice the risk of developing coronary artery disease for type A people than type B.

Stress is an element of challenge that is present in the everyday activities with which some people are confronted. Stress affects the body by increasing the serum cholesterol level. How one adapts to stressful situations is the key to the degree of body damage caused by it. Attempts should be made to minimize the amount of stress present in job-related circumstances in addition to home lifestyles.

Signs of Cardiac Arrest

Unlike the subjective symptoms experienced only by one individual, a sign is objectively visible to other people around that individual. The condition of cardiac arrest is a life threatening situation and may be recognized by the following signs of absence of circulation:
1. State of unconsciousness
2. Pulse will be absent
3. Breathing will stop
4. Pupils will be dilated
5. Skin color will be bluish

Cardiac arrest should be considered whenever a person suddenly collapses and loses consciousness. However, there are other instances that can cause a person to pass out. If he does not respond, gently shake him and shout "Are you okay? Can you hear me?" It is essential to determine if a pulse and breathing are present. If C.P.R. is applied to someone who does not need it, there is a risk of injuring the patient.

If the pulse and breathing have ceased, cardiac and respiratory arrest have occurred. It has been estimated that 45-60 seconds is required for the pupils to dilate. Checking the size of the pupils may help to determine the time of cardiac arrest. Bluish skin color is due to the lack of oxygenated blood supply to the body tissues.

Symptoms

A symptom is a subjective feeling. Pain can be described in many different ways and is greatly influenced by each individual's tolerance level to the degree of pain experienced.

People should be aware of and heed the warning signals of a heart attack. If the following symptoms are present, it is important to seek immediate medical attention. Too many lives are lost because these symptoms relating to the cardiac system are passed off as symptoms of a gastro-intestinal tract disorder.

1. Prolonged pain or unusual discomfort in the center of the chest which may travel to the shoulder, neck, jaw or back.
2. Sweating may be present.
3. Nausea and vomiting may occur.
4. A strong feeling of apprehension may persist.
5. Difficulty breathing or shortness of breath may be felt.
6. Skin color may turn pale or bluish gray.

These symptoms occur primarily because of the gradual narrowing of the coronary arteries, which results in a reduced blood supply to the heart muscles. Over 60 percent of the annual deaths from coronary artery disease are sudden deaths, usually occurring within two hours after the onset of symptoms suggesting a heart attack. This is due to a deficit in the electrical system, causing the heart to beat irregularly. These irregular rhythms are preventable and treatable if detected early, but are lethal if the person does not seek medical attention.

Therefore, the first few hours are critical and medical supervision is essential. Several reasons exist leading to a delay in seeking medical management.

1. Lack of information regarding the significance of the symptoms and the urgency for seeking immediate medical care.
2. Denial of the importance of chest discomfort due to the fear of a heart attack and its seriousness.
3. Misinterpretation of symptoms as a disorder of the gastro-intestinal tract.

4. Lack of a family physician.
5. Lack of support by family members or friends to seek medical advice.
6. Lack of knowledge to gain admission into the hospital system.

Within the past few years, numerous public educational programs have been initiated. These programs are directed towards teaching the frequent occurrence of coronary artery disease, the common early symptoms of a heart attack and the effectiveness of prompt medical care. Individuals at high risk should be identified and educated to change their lifestyles and habits.

Stages of Cardiac Arrest

Cardiac arrest is the end result of life. Too frequently its occurrence is unexpected in people who previously felt healthy and free of any symptoms of coronary artery disease. Autopsy reports have revealed that death results from dilatation of the coronary arteries and cardiac arrest. To summarize, cardiac arrest is the abrupt cessation of effective pumping activity of the heart, which causes an interruption of adequate blood supply to the body tissues for an indefinite period of time.

Death does not usually occur as a sudden and irreversible event. Actually, a timed sequence of events takes place from the moment the individual stops breathing, or his heart stops, until he is dead. Physicians refer to the separation of these two phases of the death process as clinical and biological death.

Clinical death is defined as the absence of vital signs, the cessation of breathing and heartbeat. Therefore, no pulse or blood pressure can be elicited. As determined both experimentally and clinically, the time interval between the two stages of clinical death and biological death is approximately four to six minutes. Irreversible cellular changes take place after this time. Cellular function stops and the cells die because of lack of circulation of blood and, therefore, lack of adequate oxygen. This damage is permanent.

Resuscitation is the restoration of vital signs by mechanical, physiological and pharmacological means. The application of C.P.R. during the critical time period of four to six minutes can successfully ward off biological death. Immediate restoration of the circulation of oxygenated blood is required if survival and functional recovery is to be achieved. Irreversible brain damage may result if sufficient oxygen-rich blood does not reach the brain within a few minutes.

Case Study—Cardiac Arrest

A heart attack is generally preceded by one or more warning signals such as chest pain. Too frequently, however, a heart attack occurs suddenly, silently, without a warning and can be fatal. The following case study is an illustration of a cardiac arrest.

John is a 61-year-old married man with three grown sons. He is of Italian descent and has been in relatively good health most of his life. He obtains a yearly routine physical examination by his company doctor at Commonwealth Edison. He has also been under the care and supervision of his own private family physician for treatment of high cholesterol and mild elevated blood pressure, both controlled by medication. Previous electrocardiograms were considered to be within normal limits.

Tuesday, May 10, 1977, started out in the typical work day manner—but its ending was quite atypical. While driving a company truck out to Joliet, John noticed a burning sensation in his throat and upper part of his chest. Having had no past experiences with heart attack warning signals, he attributed the discomfort to indigestion. Not realizing the seriousness of this matter, he failed to seek medical attention at a nearby hospital. Instead, he and his partner stopped for a quick cup of coffee. The discomfort subsided somewhat.

After the drive back to the Harvey plant, John collapsed while getting out of the truck. His partner recognized the signs of cardiac arrest and summoned help immediately. (All employees of Commonwealth Edison Company have taken a basic first aid course and they had completed the C.P.R. instruction course just one week prior to this incident.) Two co-workers performed mouth-to-mouth ventilation and external cardiac compression until the paramedic rescue team arrived only two minutes later. Emergency measures were administered by them and John was transported to a nearby hospital. He was rushed through the emergency room and quickly admitted to the coronary intensive care unit. Today he is back at work and leading a normal life. C.P.R. saved his life.

3
The Respiratory System

Structure

The respiratory system provides a pathway for air to enter and leave the body. Breathing is a continuous exchange of atmospheric air. The respiratory system extends from the nose, nasal passages, mouth, pharynx (throat), trachea (windpipe), and to the lungs. The internal structure of the lungs consists of the bronchial tree—bronchi, bronchioles and alveolar sacs.

In the nose, cilia are present in great abundance. Cilia are short, thin hairs lining the membranes of the nasal passages. Together, with the arteries in the nose, which lie close to the surface, they warm the air as it enters the body. The cilia are extremely sensitive and easily detect foreign bodies such as dust particles. Foreign bodies act as an irritant. To eliminate the irritating source the body responds by inducing a sneeze, forcing the particle out.

The throat is formed by the nasopharynx, the back of the nose, and the oropharynx, the back of the mouth. It is tubular in shape measuring about five inches in length and serves as the common entrance to the respiratory and digestive tracts. The tongue is a muscle used primarily to assist in moving food around in the mouth during chewing. This muscle is involuntarily held in place on the floor of the mouth. Even with the body in a lying down position the tongue is maintained on the floor of the oral cavity. Danger arises in an unconscious person (perhaps suffering from a stroke, seizure, or heart attack), as the tongue may fall

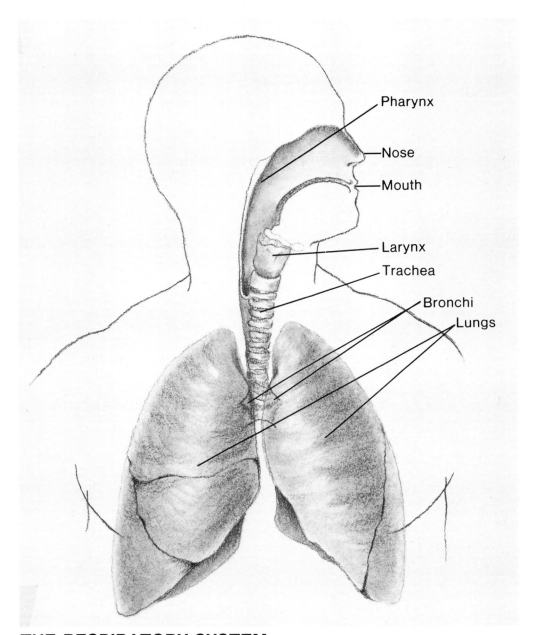

THE RESPIRATORY SYSTEM

backward in the throat blocking the windpipe and pro-
hibiting free air exchange. Caution must be exhibited
by the observer-rescuer to maintain the victim's tongue
in proper alignment to facilitate breathing. Applying
gentle upward pressure by the index fingers or thumbs
at the base of the jawbones will elevate the lower jaw.
This elevation will force the adjacent muscles connecting the tongue to maintain its normal anatomical position and alleviate the obstruction of the passageway.

The larynx, or voice box, is located at the upper end of the windpipe. It is located at the level of the Adam's apple and contains the vocal cords. Speech is attained as the air passing over the vocal cords creates a vibration resulting in phonation and articulation. The tra-

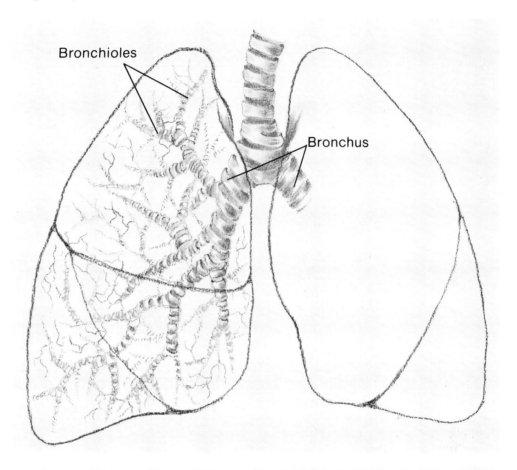

**INTERNAL
STRUCTURES
OF THE
LUNGS**

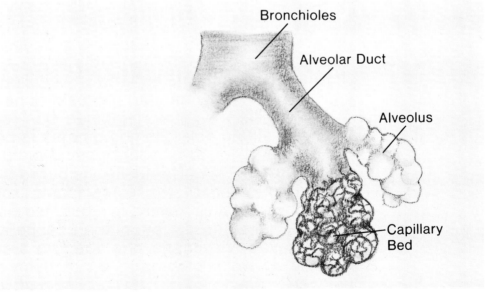

chea extends from the larynx to the bronchi. It is a flexible, cylindrical tube measuring about four and one-half inches in length and one inch in diameter. It lies in front of the esophagus and extends from the neck into the chest where it divides into two bronchi leading into the lungs.

The left bronchus is narrower but longer than the right, measuring almost two inches in length. The right bronchus is wider but shorter than the left with a length of about one inch. It also lies straighter in the right lung. For this reason, foreign bodies that have slipped into the windpipe usually lodge in the right lung. As the bronchi descend further into the lungs they branch off into smaller segments, bronchioles. Located at the end of the bronchioles lie sac-like structures, alveolae. It is here that internal breathing takes place. Oxygen from the alveoli enters the capillary bed of the pulmonary circulation and carbon dioxide leaves the blood. Oxygenated blood then returns to the left side of the heart to be circulated to the body tissues. The structure formed by the windpipe, bronchi and bronchioles resembles a tree, and therefore, is referred to as the bronchial tree.

Surrounding the bronchial tree, the lungs occupy the vast majority of space in the thoracic cage. The right and left lungs are separated by the heart. Each lung is conical in shape, of a spongy consistency and together they weigh approximately 42 ounces. The right lung is slightly heavier, broader and larger than the left, having three segments, upper, lower and middle lobes. Only two lobes, upper and lower form the left lung and its smaller size is due to the space occupied by the heart in the left side of the thorax. The uppermost portion of each lung is known as the apex. The lower portion forms the base and it lies on the diaphragm. Each lung is surrounded by a thin, moist, delicate membrane called the pleura, which covers the outer surface of the lungs and also lines the inner surface of the thorax.

The thorax is the portion of the body extending from the base of the neck to the diaphragm containing the lungs. The thoracic cavity is surrounded by the rib cage, which is expandable yet strong and provides protection for these vital organs. There are twelve pairs of ribs. The upper ten pairs curve around the sides of the body and join the sternum. The lower two pairs of ribs are called floating ribs as they are not connected to the breastbone. The ribs are held together by the intercostal muscles. The diaphragm is a gently curved dome-shaped muscle which forms the floor of the thorax, separating it from the organs found in the abdominal cavity. It is attached to the lateral, outside walls of the thorax. The sternum provides support for the anterior portion of the thoracic framework. The spinal column provides support to the posterior aspect as the backbone. Contraction and expansion of the thoracic cage are accomplished by the action of the intercostal muscles and the downward movement of the diaphragm.

Mechanics of Breathing

Breathing consists of two phases: inspiration and expiration. Inspiration takes place as the air enters the respiratory system and expiration takes place as the air leaves the body and is returned to the environment.

Actually there are two types of breathing that occur in the human body simultaneously. External breathing is the movement of air from the atmosphere through the respiratory tract. It is visually observed as the chest wall expands and rises. Internal breathing cannot be seen. It is the gaseous exchange of oxygen and carbon dioxide within the air sacs of the lungs and is frequently referred to as cellular respirations.

External breathing consists of two phases: inspiration and expiration. The movement of air into and out of the respiratory tract is controlled by the muscles surrounding the rib cage and the *diaphragm,* a dome-shaped muscle that forms the floor of the thoracic cage. It normally curves upward in the relaxed position. As it contracts, the curved portions become flattened or even curved downward. The space in the thoracic cage is enlarged. During inspiration the muscles between the ribs contract causing an elevation of the chest wall. The diameter of the thoracic cavity increases; thus the lungs inflate or expand and enlarge.

Expiration occurs as the diaphragm relaxes, and the curved sides return to their normal upward position. Simultaneously, the muscles surrounding the ribs relax, decreasing the diameter of the thoracic cage. The lungs contract or somewhat deflate causing expiration.

Function

Oxygen is one of the basic needs of the human body. A constant source is required to maintain life. Oxygen is readily available, but can be absorbed only through the lungs. The function of the respiratory system is to remove oxygen from the air, transport it to the cells, and eliminate carbon dioxide, an end-product of cellular metabolism, from the body back to the atmosphere. This task is accomplished by *pulmonary ventilation,* exchange of gases within the lungs and the pulmonary circulation.

The alveoli of the bronchial tree and the capillary bed of the circulatory system lie together in close proximity. Venous blood, having a high carbon dioxide content and a low oxygen content, is brought to the lungs by one of the pulmonary arteries. The carbon dioxide travels from the capillary bed through the alveolar membrane into the alveolar sac and is released into the atmosphere during expiration. In exchange for the carbon dioxide, oxygen is retrieved from the alveoli and travels across the capillary membrane into the pulmonary circulation. Now the gaseous content of the blood has been reversed, with a high oxygen content and low carbon dioxide content. One of the pulmonary veins returns the blood to the left side of the heart for circulation to the body tissues. As metabolism occurs, the arterial blood releases oxygen to the cells and retrieves carbon dioxide. This venous blood returns to the right side of the heart and is pumped to the lungs for replenishment.

Inspired air is composed of 21 percent oxygen, 79 percent nitrogen and 0.4 percent carbon dioxide. These amounts readily supply sufficient oxygen to meet the body needs of an adult during rest or exercise. Expired air still has a high percentage of oxygen, approximately 16 percent, but carbon dioxide has increased to 4 percent and nitrogen content has remained unchanged. Artificial ventilation by the mouth-to-mouth or mouth-to-nose technique delivers an adequate amount of oxygen to the victim. In fact, expired air, high in carbon dioxide, that enters the victim's respiratory system acts as a stimulant to induce spontaneous breathing. As the carbon dioxide content builds up in the blood, the control center of the brain, the *medulla,* is triggered off to re-induce breathing. Blood high in carbon dioxide and low in oxygen influences an increase in pulmonary ventilation. Likewise, ventilation is decreased with an increased oxygen and decreased carbon dioxide blood level.

These gaseous levels are determined by obtaining a sample of blood from the arterial circulation, and are referred to as arterial blood gases. In the critical care unit of a hospital these blood gas levels are carefully monitored by physicians and nurses. The oxygen and carbon dioxide levels in the blood indicate whether or not there is adequate tissue oxygenation. Other indications of adequate oxygen supply to body tissue can be visually observed by checking the color of the lips and nailbeds. Normally they are pink in color.

Hemoglobin is an iron and protein compound carried by the red blood cells that combines with oxygen. It acts as a transporter carrying oxygen to the cells. It is this hemoglobin structure, bound to the oxygen molecule, that gives blood its rich red color. If the lips or nailbeds appear somewhat bluish, the oxygen level will be low and oxygen will need to be administered.

Control of Breathing

The respiratory control center is located in the medulla, a section of the brain. Breathing is spontaneous and controlled involuntarily during coughing, speaking, swallowing and laughing. The rate and depth of each breath is affected by three factors: the carbon dioxide content of the blood, the oxygen content and exercise. The most influential stimulus is the carbon dioxide content of the blood. When the carbon dioxide level rises above normal, both the rate and depth of breathing is increased.

The rate and rhythm of breathing is controlled by the medulla in the brain. At rest, the respiratory rate ranges between 16-20 per minute. Inspiration takes approximately two seconds; because expiration is normally a passive process (not controlled consciously), it usually requires approximately three seconds. Heavy exercise can increase the respiratory rate ten to twenty times. The rate increases proportionately to meet the oxygen demands of the body tissues. Excitement, fear, and pain also raise the respiratory rate as well as the heart rate.

The rhythm is usually classified as regular, if it takes place in even intervals. However, alterations in rate and rhythm can occur. *Hyperventilation* is an increase in ventilation in excess of the amount required to maintain normal arterial blood oxygen and carbon dioxide levels. It can be caused by anxiety, fever, bacterial infections, low blood pressure, and pain. Hyperventilation is characterized by rapid, shallow respirations. The time interval is decreased in both the inspiratory and expiratory phases. *Hypoventilation* exists when an insufficient volume of air enters the lungs each minute relative to the metabolic activity of the body. It can be caused by depression of the respiratory center due to general anesthesia, excess narcotics, limitation of lung movement, pulmonary diseases, tumor, or pneumonia. Hypoventilation is characterized by slow, deep breaths. The carbon dioxide is not completely blown off, and the residual builds up in the blood causing an excess of carbon dioxide and insufficient oxygen content of the blood.

Dyspnea is a medical term used to describe difficulty breathing and is usually described by the person experiencing it as shortness of breath or in terms such as, ''I can't seem to catch my breath.'' This abnormality frequently follows some type of physical activity such as climbing several flights of stairs. *Orthopnea* is a more specific term used to label difficulty breathing during the night. The difficulty breathing is generally due to the sleeping position. Many people must sleep propped up with several pillows to maintain an almost sitting position before the shortness of breath somewhat subsides.

Apnea is a term used synonymously with respiratory arrest and means the cessation of respirations. *Cheyne-stokes* breathing is a combination of hypoventilation and periods of apnea. This grossly irregular pattern of breathing is readily observed in a dying person.

Sometimes the body adjusts the rate and rhythm to compensate for a metabolic disturbance in an attempt to return the body to a state of equilibrium.

Lung Capacity

Pulmonary function studies have been devised to determine the capacity of the lungs. The tests are performed by blowing air into a machine called a *bronchospirometer,* that records the volumes on a moving piece of graphic paper. Volumes differ between females and males due to body size and physical development. Body surface area of females is less, therefore, the total volume of inspired air will be less than that of the male.

With each normal breath approximately 500 milliliters (ml.) of air is moved in and out of the lungs. This measurement represents the tidal volume. With forced inspiration approximately 3000 ml. of air enters above the 500 ml. tidal volume and is called the inspiratory reserve volume. Expiratory reserve volume is the amount of air forcefully expired following normal breathing and is usually about 1100 ml. Residual volume is the volume of air that remains in the lungs at the end of maximal expiration, 1200 ml.

Inspiratory capacity, 3500 ml., is the combination of

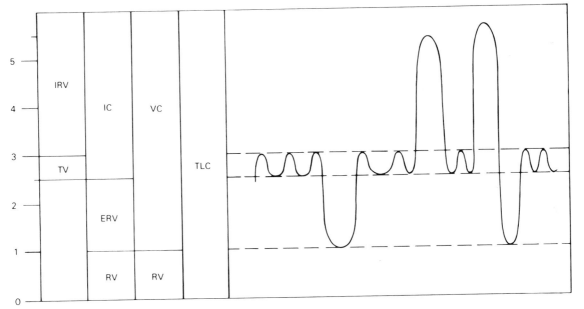

LUNG CAPACITY

IRV—Inspiratory Reserve Volume
TV—Tidal Volume
ERV—Expiratory Reserve Volume
RV—Residual Volume

IC—Inspiratory Capacity
VC—Vital Capacity
TLC—Total Lung Capacity

tidal volume and inspiratory reserve volume. Vital capacity is the sum of inspiratory capacity and expiratory reserve volume, approximately 4000 ml. It is the maximal amount of air that can be expired with force, following forced maximal inspiration. The total lung capacity, 5800 ml., is the volume of air contained in the lungs at the end of a maximal inspiration. It is the sum of all volumes.

These volumes represent the functional ability of the lungs. Low measurements may be caused by several factors; limitation of lung movement due to such conditions as pneumonia, tumor or asthma; or by restrictive conditions of the muscles causing a limitation of movement of the thoracic cage.

These volumes aid the physician in formulating a diagnosis and developing a treatment plan. If symptoms are present, the individual must recognize what activities cause the difficulty breathing; he must learn to adapt his lifestyle within these limitations.

Irritants and Obstructions

Energy is required for the expansion of the thoracic cage by the muscles surrounding the ribs. Normally there exists a small amount of airway resistance, but the amount of energy needed to move the air along the passages is slight. However, the energy required to move air in and out greatly increases in proportion to the increased airway resistance due to obstructions of the airway caused by conditions such as asthma or obstructive emphysema. Irritants such as nicotine from cigarette smoke cause a temporary constriction of the air passages. Dust particles and pollens have the same effect on a person having allergies or asthma. A wheezing sound may accompany breathing.

Normal expirations are considered passive. During exercise, expirations change to strong, forceful acts. Muscles around the ribs actually pull the chest downward forcing the diaphragm upward. In addition to accommodating the body's increased demands for oxygen, forced expiration is also utilized to expel foreign objects from the respiratory passages. A cough is induced as the *epiglottis,* the gatekeeper of the respiratory and digestive tracts located in the windpipe, remains closed while the expiratory muscles are vigorously contracted. The air within the lower base of the lungs is temporarily prevented from leaving the lungs. This causes the pressure to build up. The glottis suddenly opens and a blast of air rushes through the windpipe ejecting any foreign object which may have been lodged.

Case Study—Respiratory Arrest

Respiratory arrest is directly related to other factors. Ingestion of drugs, especially medications containing narcotics, have a depressant effect on the respiratory control center, the medulla. Severe allergic reactions to some drugs such as penicillin can result in cessation of breathing. Other causes of respiratory arrest are choking, drowning, smoke inhalation, carbon monoxide poisoning and cardiac arrest. Respiratory arrest is a gradual process. The following case study will illustrate the phases.

Clyde is a 64-year-old male who entered the hospital with a diagnosis of pneumonia and malnutrition. He was grossly underweight, and medical and nursing care was directed toward the latter problem of building his weight back up to normal. He was placed on a high protein, high caloric diet. But his appetite was poor. He was started on intravenous feedings in addition to his diet. Eventually he was placed on high nutritional intravenous feedings and gastric tube feedings because his oral intake of food and fluids was inadequate to sustain life.

At first, Clyde had mild difficulty breathing, usually associated with physical activity. Later the difficulty breathing became severe even while at rest. Eating was too strenuous. Eventually his breathing became shallow and quite labored. A low carbon dioxide concentration caused depression of the respiratory center, resulting in progressively longer periods of breathlessness/apnea. Breathing ceased altogether and cardiac arrest followed within minutes.

Mouth-to-mouth ventilation and external cardiac compression was initiated immediately, and Clyde was transferred to the intensive care unit and placed on a ventilator, a machine which takes over the breathing process until the underlying problem is resolved and normal breathing resumes. C.P.R. saved his life.

4
The Uses of C.P.R.

Before learning how to perform C.P.R., it is essential to know when life support measures are needed. As previously described, the most frequent application for C.P.R. techniques is in the treatment of heart attack victims. Other instances, whereby sudden cessation of life resulting from cardiac arrest and/or respiratory arrest should be followed with the immediate administration of C.P.R. measures, follow.

Electrocution

Priorities must be set in the case of electrocution. It is imperative that the source of the electrical current is shut off before any rescue attempt is made. Do not attempt to pull the victim away from the electric wire if he is still in contact, but instead push or pull the source of electricity away from the victim with a nonconductive material such as a piece of wood, rolled paper, sheet, or blanket. Rescue attempts would prove fatal to the rescuer when extremely high voltage electrical cables are involved, as it takes a long time for the electric company to locate and then turn off the power source. One cannot take the risk that the power has been turned off, and by that time, the victim is beyond revival. With electrocution, burns will be present at the point of entry and exit, but the first priority is to restore breathing and circulation.

Smoke Inhalation

Smoke inhalation and carbon monoxide poisoning occur in a small area that quickly accumulates the gaseous fumes. If possible, quickly remove the victim from the source of gas or smoke into a safe environment. If breathing has already failed, mouth-to-mouth resucitation must be initiated immediately. If the victim cannot be moved, attempt to cut off the source. Open windows and doors to allow fresh air to enter the enclosed area. Since gaseous fumes and smoke rise, keep the victim close to the ground. Quick action is essential; after four minutes the oxygen supply to the brain is significantly lowered and damage occurs.

Drugs

Respiratory complications and failure may result from drug ingestion, the most obvious condition being an overdose, either accidental or intentional, of pills containing narcotic substances. The combined effects of several drugs can result in depression of the respiratory center causing breathing to become so slowed and irregular in pattern that it may cease entirely. Other causes of respiratory arrest can be severe allergic reactions to such drugs as penicillin or an adverse or undesirable effect to a drug. The situation must be assessed quickly and artificial ventilation initiated immediately and maintained until the victim begins to breathe on his own, or until he can be transported to a facility where mechanical ventilatory assistance is available.

Automobile Accidents

In a serious automobile accident, victims can be knocked unconscious and cardiac and respiratory functions endangered. First aid should be directed towards maintaining these life support systems until paramedic rescue teams arrive at the scene.

Drowning

In the United States, 10 percent of all accidental deaths each year are caused by drownings, claiming about 8000 lives. Drowning usually occurs when an individual is not able to stay afloat due to fatigue, lack of skill in swimming, panic, or encountering some acute medical problem while the individual is in or near the water, such as an epileptic seizure or a heart attack.

Treatment is the same as for other causes of cardiac arrest. Mouth-to-mouth resuscitation is more difficult due to a fine froth from air passages. Frequently, time is wasted trying to drain water from lungs, and clearing the mouth of sand, seaweed, and artificial dentures. Most recently reported, yet still in the experimental stages, the Heimlich maneuver has been successfully used to revive drowning victims when mouth-to-mouth resuscitation had failed. This technique will be discussed in the next chapter.

Choking

Choking is most frequently encountered during eating and involves a piece of meat, bread, or foreign object. Usually a sharp pat between the shoulder blades is sufficient to resolve the situation. Occasionally, a foreign body becomes lodged in the throat causing extreme distress. A child can be held head down and given several sharp slaps on the back. The same treatment can be given to an adult except that his head should be placed between his knees. If this fails, and breathing ceases, mouth-to-mouth resuscitation will have to be attempted. If the air will not pass down, extend the victim's head, open the mouth and use anything (i.e., fingers, tongs, etc.) to attempt to dislodge the object and remove it, if it can be seen. In the past, if a physician were available, a *tracheotomy,* an incision in the trachea, was performed to allow passage of air. For removal of objects not visible, the Heimlich maneuver will be discussed next.

5
Heimlich Maneuver

In the United States, an average of 3900 healthy individuals strangle each year because food or foreign objects become lodged in the back of the throat obstructing the airway, or windpipe. Fatalities from food choking, the sixth leading cause of accidental death, can be totally avoided through a lifesaving technique known as the Heimlich maneuver. Dr. Henry J. Heimlich of Cincinnati, Ohio, first attempted this technique on beagles in 1974. Its success on animals prompted his article in *Emergency Medicine* which later reached the news media including newspapers, radio, television stations and several leading women's magazines, informing both the medical and general public of its use and success.

As cited in numerous replies to his article, the scope of its use included a variety of settings: a family dwelling, banquet, diner, cocktail party, hospital, garden party, and beach where a lifeguard rescued a drowning victim.

Because death occurs suddenly within 4-6 minutes, action must be initiated quickly. Physicians who have previously provided appropriate medical treatment by performing a tracheotomy (opening through the neck into the trachea) have refrained from doing so after successfully saving a life by utilizing the Heimlich maneuver. Physicians, nurses and other medical personnel are not usually present to perform lifesaving measures. Recently, an instrument has been devised for extracting food from the back of the throat, but the double limitations of the instrument's availability and the presence of someone possessing the knowledge of how to use it is a rare coincidence outside of a hospital. Therefore, a first aid procedure that does not require specialized instruments or equipment and can be performed by any informed layman is necessary to save people from food asphyxiation.

Signs

Food choking occurs quickly and without warning. The victim cannot breathe or speak; his skin color becomes pale, then bluish, and then he collapses to the floor. The circumstances surrounding the incident have caused experts to call it a cafe coronary. The episode is often confused with a heart attack, although a heart attack victim usually verbalizes his symptoms, which occur over a longer period of time. Signs of a heart attack also include profuse sweating, chest pain and nausea—signs that are not present at the time of airway obstruction.

Food choking occurs during the disruption of the synchronized process of breathing in air, inspiration, and swallowing of food. Occurring simultaneously instead, the food is held tightly against the opening of the voice box with suction imitating that of a vacuum cleaner. Attempts to clear the obstruction, administering mouth-to-mouth resuscitation will prove unsuccessful, and the effort will waste precious seconds. The technique of the Heimlich maneuver breaks the suction.

Since food asphyxiation occurs during inspiration, the lungs are expanded. Pressing one's fist upward in the abdomen above the navel, but below the rib cage, elevates the diaphragm. Sudden elevation of the diaphragm compresses the lungs within the boundaries of the rib cage increasing the air pressure, forcing it out through the windpipe. Along with the air, the food or foreign object will be ejected, thus alleviating the obstructed airway.

Technique: Rescuer Standing

Stand behind the victim, wrap arms around his waist. Grasp the fist of one hand with the other hand, placing the thumb side of the fist against the victim's abdomen. Hand placement need not be precise, but must be

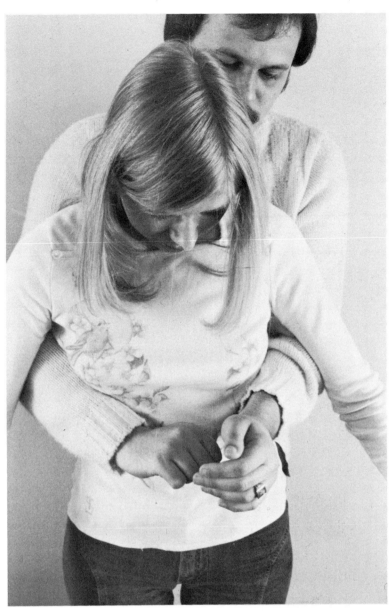

At left, rescuer standing behind victim.

Thumb side of fist, below.

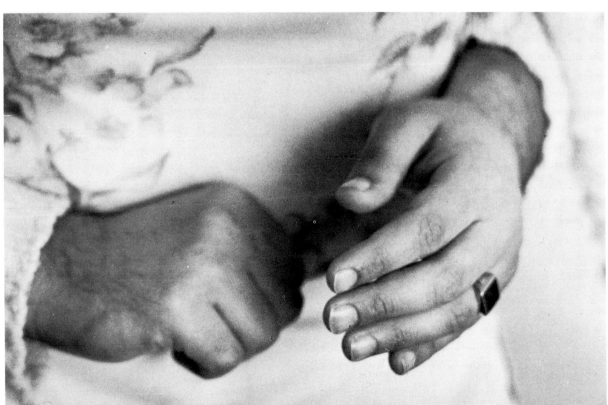

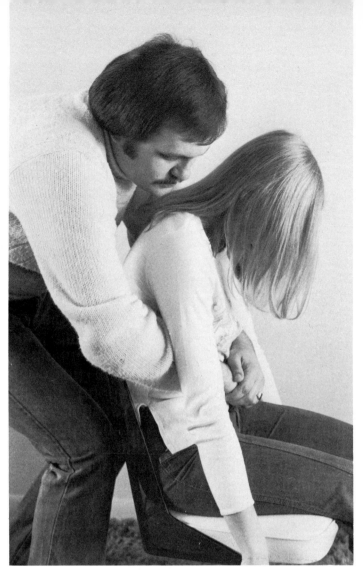

Victim sitting.

slightly above the navel and below the rib cage. With a quick, upward thrust, the fist is pressed into the victim's abdomen. If necessary, the technique is repeated several times. Since choking occurs most frequently while sitting at a table, the rescuer may need to approach the victim as he is still seated, from behind, and perform the maneuver in the same manner, but with knees slightly bent to gain leverage.

Technique: Rescuer Kneeling

Occasionally the victim will collapse to the floor. The rescuer should kneel on the floor, facing the victim, straddling his hips. Place the heel of one hand on the victim's abdomen slightly above the navel and below the rib cage. The second hand is placed on top of the bottom hand. With a quick upward thrust, pressure is applied into the victim's abdomen, and repeated sever-

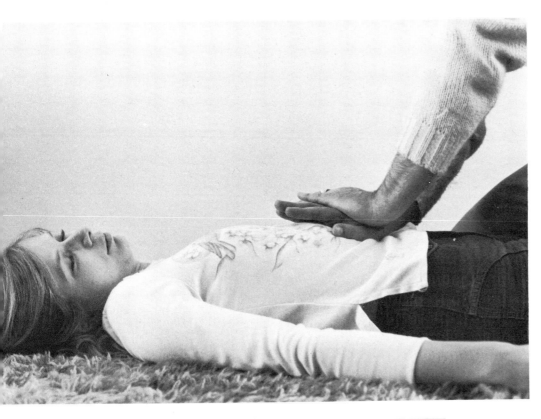

Victim lying down, above.

At left, rescuer straddling victim.

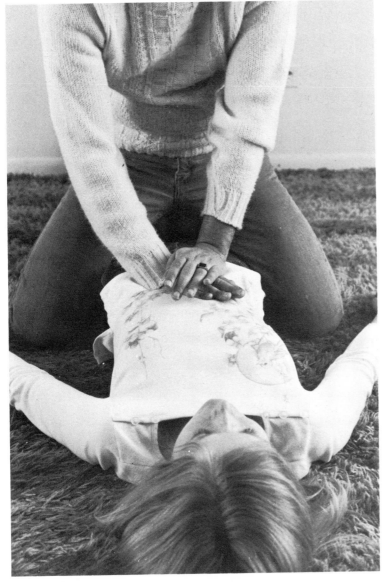

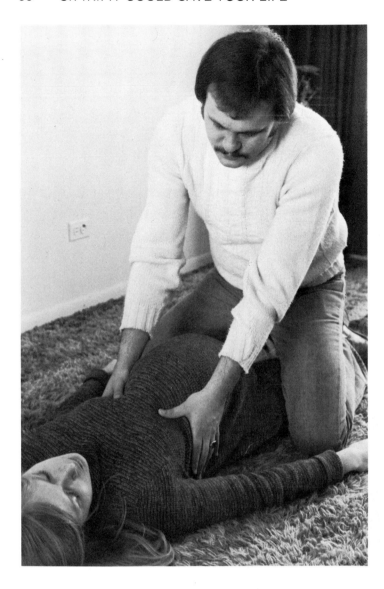

Variation for applying maneuver to a pregnant woman.

al times. Pressure on the abdomen may cause recently consumed food to be expelled. If vomiting occurs, quickly place the victim on his side and wipe out his mouth.

With improper application of the Heimlich maneuver, complications can occur. If pressure is applied to the ribs, fractures are possible. Pressure applied by the arms to the sides of the victim rather than the fists to the abdomen can cause injury to organs such as the liver and spleen. Performing the maneuver on a pregnant woman may injure the baby, but will at least save the mother's life. With spread fingers the hands are placed along the lower aspect of the rib cage. Pressure is concentrated on the heels of the hands and applied in the same inward, upward manner.

6
C.P.R. Techniques

In 1974, the National Conference on Cardio-Pulmonary Resuscitation and Emergency Coronary Care developed standards of C.P.R. There is a simple formula for providing emergency care, which has become known as the *ABC's* and consists of *Airway, Breathing and Circulation.* If quickly initiated, resuscitative measures will save the victim's life.

The victim will be unable to breathe unless the nasal passages and mouth are clear from foreign objects that may obstruct or block air entering or leaving the lungs. If artificial dentures or food are blocking the mouth or throat, they must be removed. Occasionally, mucous or vomitus will collect in the oral cavity and can be removed by wiping the mouth with a clean cloth. If a foreign object is causing the obstruction, the object can be forced out by using the Heimlich maneuver which has been discussed previously.

A: Airway

If breathing has ceased, the victim must be placed on a flat, firm surface, lying supine on his back. The floor or ground is preferred, as it is easily accessible and provides a firm supportive surface not attained by placing a person on a sofa, couch, or mattress. The rescuer must assume a kneeling position to the right side of the victim. The tongue, which is also a muscle, tends to roll backward in the throat to block the windpipe, obstructing airflow. The rescuer must hold the victim's head in such a position as to alleviate this po-

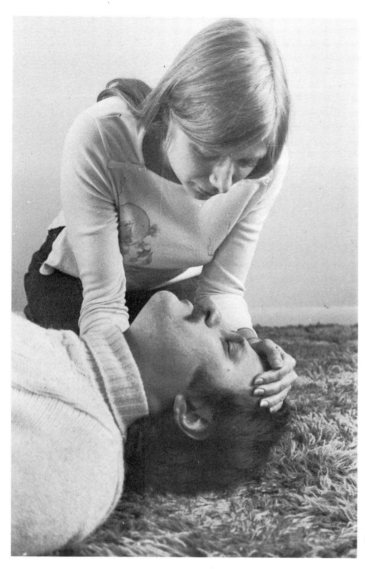

Opening airway and maintaining proper head alignment.

tential blockage. This is achieved by placing the right hand under the victim's neck and gently pushing upward. The left hand is placed on his forehead exerting gentle pressure downward. By supporting the victim's head in proper alignment, the tongue is maintained in an elevated position conducive to the movement of air both in and out of the lungs.

The airway should be open now, and breathing may begin spontaneously, exhibited by a rising movement of the chest wall. In addition to observing for chest movement, an ear placed close to the victim's nose and mouth will detect any faint noises of breathing or actually allow the warm air exchange taking place to be felt. If there is no breathing, artificial ventilation by the mouth-to-mouth or mouth-to-nose method must be initiated immediately.

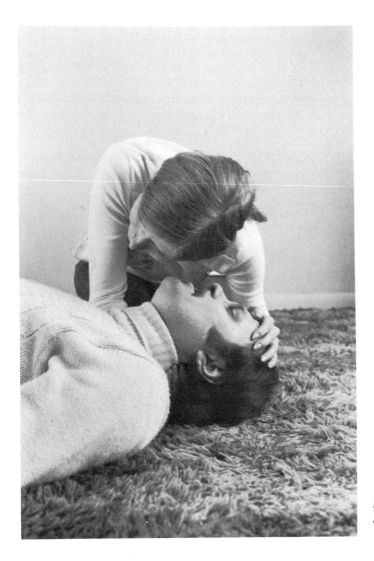

Looking, listening, and feeling for air exchange.

B: Breathing
(Mouth-to-Mouth Resuscitation)

The arm lift/back pressure, an old method of restoring breathing, has been replaced by the mouth-to-mouth technique, as it is the easiest and most efficient way to assist in breathing for someone else. An individual who has ceased to breathe must be given artificial respiration by instilling air to his mouth or nose immediately. As mentioned earlier, the rescuer's left hand is already resting on the victim's forehead with the palm exerting slight downward pressure. The nostrils are gently pinched together between the thumb and index finger of the left hand to prevent any air leakage. An airtight seal is formed as the rescuer places his lips firmly

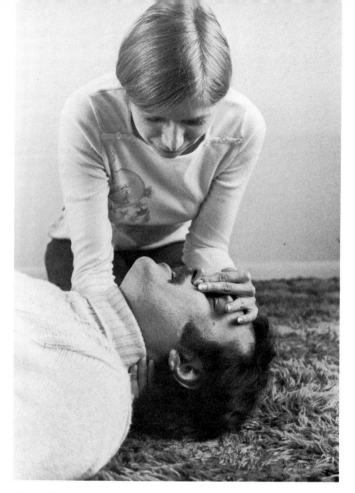

Pinching the nostrils to prevent air leakage.

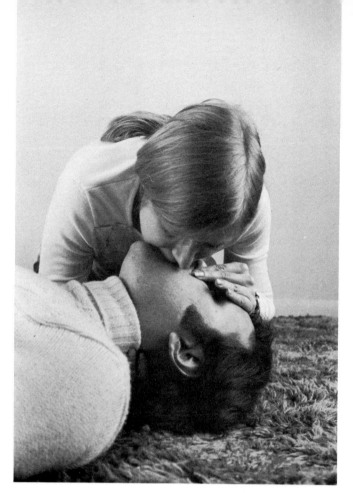

Airtight seal for mouth-to-mouth ventilation.

around the victim's mouth. With forceful exhalation, air is pushed into the victim's lungs causing them to expand and, therefore, causing the rising movement of the chest wall. The rescuer's head is twisted slightly for ease in observing the rising chest movement and listening for air exchange, indications of adequate ventilation. The seal must be broken momentarily to allow the person to exhale and to allow the rescuer to take in another deep breath in preparation for administering another artificial ventilation.

Normal respiratory rate ranges between 16 and 22 per minute. Like the pulse rate, the respiratory rate increases with exercise due to an increased demand for oxygen. While the body is at rest, breathing may decrease to even twelve per minute, because the oxygen requirement is lowered. During artificial ventilation, four breaths are given initially to allow adequate ventilation for a period of fifteen seconds. The minimal requirement of the body at rest must be maintained by the rescuer while performing resuscitative measures.

Therefore, respirations are delivered at approximately twelve per minute.

Room air that we normally breathe contains 21 percent oxygen. The oxygen content of the exhaled air that enters the victim's lungs is approximately 75 percent that of normal room air, or 16 percent, and is sufficient enough to maintain adequate body tissue oxygenation and prevention of brain damage. The carbon dioxide content of victim's forced inspiration serves to stimulate his own respiratory center, since the most potent stimulus to breathing is a high build up of carbon dioxide in the blood. The procedure is continued until either breathing starts spontaneously or mechanical breathing assistance becomes available.

C: Circulation
(External Cardiac Compression)

If unexpected cardiac arrest occurs, the ABC's of emergency care are required and must be administered in rapid sequence. As previously discussed, the heart is located between the sternum and spinal column. As sufficient pressure is applied to the sternum, it is depressed. This will squeeze the heart forcing its blood contents into the circulation. Releasing the pressure momentarily will allow it to refill in preparation for another compression.

Placement of the hands and timing are the most important aspects of external cardiac compression. A few landmarks must be established before attempting to maintain artificial circulation. The heart is located at approximately the level of the fifth rib and may be easily identified on an unclothed, thin person. An imaginary line connecting the nipples will also provide a guideline. The lowermost tip of the sternum is called the *xiphoid process,* a thin sword-shaped piece of bone that protrudes slightly. Pressure at this point must be avoided as it may be injured easily. After locating the xiphoid process with the index and middle fingers of the right hand, the heel of the left hand is placed firmly on the chest wall next to the fingers of the right hand towards the victim's head. This is the precise site of cardiac compression, two fingerbreadths, about one and one-half inches above the tip of the sternum. The heel of the right hand is then placed on top of the left hand

and the fingers are interlocked to keep them off the chest wall. When properly placed, the heel of the left hand will feel the firm, flat surface of the sternum.

To provide adequate artificial circulation, the sternum must be depressed one and one-half to two inches. This is not an easy task and can become tiring to the rescuer if not performed efficiently. Approximately 80-100 pounds of pressure is required to achieve the sternal depression. While maintaining a kneeling position close to the victim's body next to his right side, most of the rescuer's body weight must be shifted to his or her hands. The shoulders must be directly above the victim's body at a 90 degree angle with the arms straight and elbows locked.

The normal heart rate ranges between 60 and 100 beats per minute. Exercise will increase the rate and rest will decrease it. Therefore, chest compressions are delivered at a rate of one per second, or about 60 compressions per minute, which is the body's requirement to sustain adequate circulation. The compressions must be carried out in a smooth, rhythmical, and uninterrupted pattern. The heels of the rescuer's hands

Locating the xiphoid process.

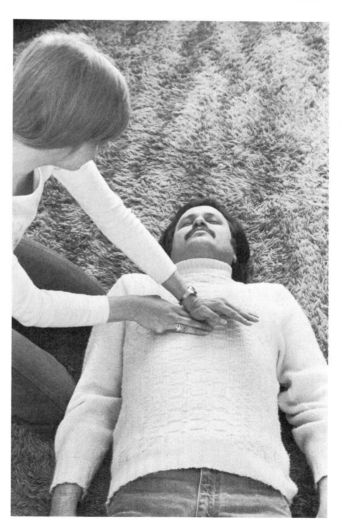

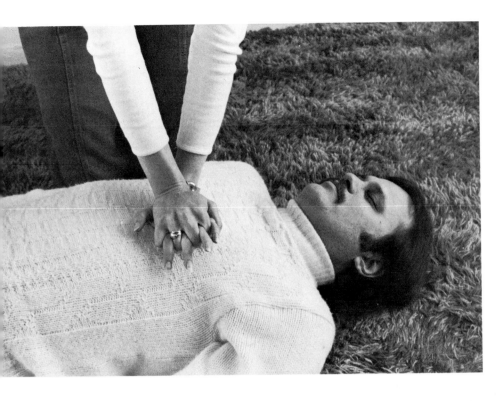

*Finding the
pressure point.*

*Proper hand placement—fingers interlocked,
elbows straight.*

*Rescuer's shoulders directly over victim's chest
at a 90-degree angle.*

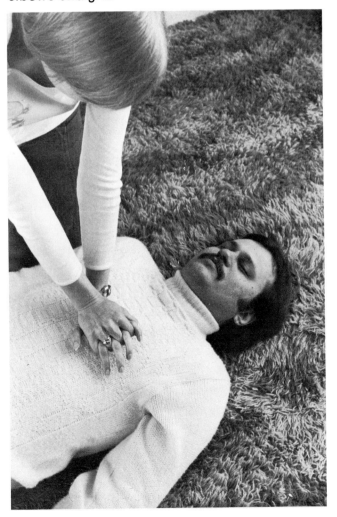

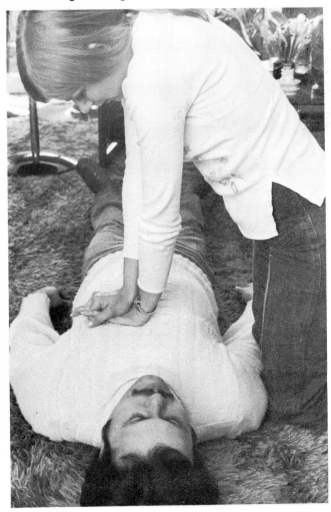

should not be removed from the chest wall between compressions, but pressure should be completely released to allow the sternum to return to a normal resting position. This split-second resting phase allows the heart chambers to fill in preparation for another compression.

C.P.R. can be performed by one person alone and the description of hand placement has been described for those circumstances. The technique obviously is less tiresome if carried out by two persons. In this instance, the rescuers will find it easier to work opposite from each other necessitating hand placement to be reversed. The person performing external cardiac compression is usually designated as the captain of the

C.P.R. by two rescuers.

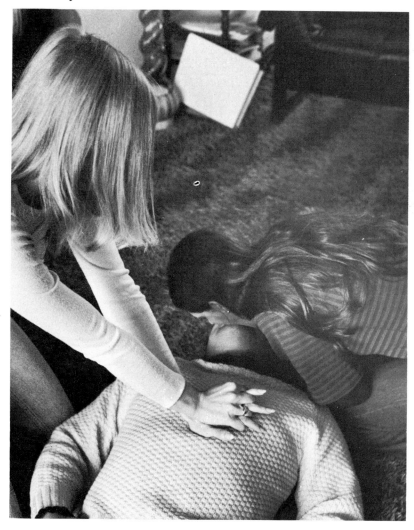

team and counts the compressions aloud to coordinate the ventilations to be delivered in a rhythmical pattern. Proper timing is achieved by counting one 1000, one 2000, one 3000, one 4000, one 5000. The heart is compressed on each count of one; pressure is released on the thousand count. At the count of 5000, a ventilation is delivered without interruption of the cycle.

Resuscitation by one rescuer is initiated by delivering four quick ventilations, then requires a repetitious cycle of 15 compressions followed by two ventilations. C.P.R. administered by two rescuers is initiated by delivering two quick ventilations, then a repetitious cycle consisting of five compressions followed by one ventilation. The rescuers must work together as a team. If one person becomes fatigued, they may switch positions. The person performing artificial respiration moves to the side of the victim immediately after he has inflated the lungs. He places his hands in the proper position and takes over cardiac compressions between the counts of 2000 and 3000. The rescuer who has been compressing then moves to the head and administers the next breath on the count of 5000.

If administered properly, the results of effective cardio-pulmonary resuscitation will be evidenced by measuring a pulse on the neck approximately one inch to either side of the Adam's apple and should be checked periodically. Another indication of efficient administration of C.P.R. is the pupillary reaction to light. Constriction of the pupils in response to light indicates there is an adequate supply of oxygenated blood being circulated to the brain cells.

It is difficult to estimate eighty pounds of pressure, and this requires a great deal of practice at home in addition to application on life-sized mannequins in a formal classroom setting. Two fairly firm sofa cushions stacked and placed on the floor will simulate the depth of an individual's body while lying in a supine position. With the heels of the hand in proper position, the hard surface of the floor should be detected. An easier and more accurate method is to use the bathroom scale. This exercise is not easy but is attainable with frequent practice and should be prior knowledge rather than guess work when the application is essential during actual resuscitation of a victim.

Complications to the victim result from improper positioning of the rescuer's hands. Rib fractures may occur when the fingers of the rescuer's hands exert pressure on the ribs. This complication can be avoided by interlocking the fingers of both hands and exerting pressure on the chest wall by placing the body weight on the heels of the hands alone. Injury to the xiphoid process of the sternum can be prevented by first locating the xiphoid process and proper positioning of the hands approximately one and one-half inches above it. Proper hand placement minimizes possible lacerations to the liver or spleen.

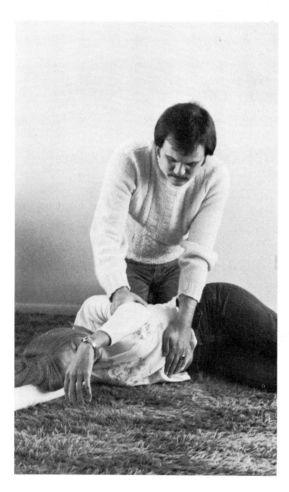

Relieving gastric distention.

Artificial breathing can cause gastric distention, particularly with airway obstruction. Severe distention may be dangerous because it exerts upward pressure on the diaphragm and restricts the space normally occupied by the expanding lungs during inspiration. To reduce the gastric distention, C.P.R. must be briefly interrupted. The victim should be rolled onto his side to facilitate drainage of stomach contents as the rescuer places gentle but firm pressure on the victim's abdomen between the navel and the rib cage. Then C.P.R. should be continued. The possible complications resulting from cardio-pulmonary resuscitation are far outweighed by the alternative the victim faces if resuscitation is not performed.

Variations for Administering C.P.R. to a Child or Infant

When resuscitating a child or infant, C.P.R. must be administered with a few variations. The weight and body surface is much less than the adult and, therefore, requires less force and effort on the part of the rescuer. Yet C.P.R. must be delivered based on the victim's body needs.

The heartbeat of the infant normally can range up to 140 beats per minute. And the range for an older child is usually between 80-100 beats per minute. Therefore, to meet their minimal requirements, external cardiac compression is delivered at a rate of approximately 80-100 per minute. The anatomical structure differs slightly as the ventricles of the heart lie higher in the chest wall. Pressure must be applied at the middle of the sternum for both infants and small children. Using the index and middle fingers gently to depress the sternum one-half to three-quarters of an inch is sufficient pressure for maintaining effective artificial circulation of an infant. Only the heel of one hand is required to depress the child's sternum three-quarters to one and one-half inches. The compression rate for a child is 80-100 per minute.

The respiratory rate is faster for the infant and child because there is a lesser capacity of the lungs. The amount of air delivered must be adjusted to the individual's capacity for expansion based on the size and body surface of that person. Small breaths of air are exhaled into the mouth of the child. The rescuer may choose to form an airtight seal over the infant's nose and mouth to deliver small puffs of air while administering artificial ventilation to the infant.

Extension of the neck and head must be done carefully as the tissues are quite pliable in small children and infants. Hyperextension of the head alone may obstruct the airway. C.P.R. is delivered at a faster rate of one ventilation every three seconds, or 20 per minute. Tilting the head backward raises the victim's back from the firm supporting surface. Placing a rolled towel or blanket between the shoulder blades will provide the needed support.

In the case of a small infant, one hand under the back with the head resting on the forearm in a cradle-like fashion will maintain the infant in proper alignment.

If airway obstruction of a small child is evident, quickly invert the child's head downward supporting his body weight. With the heel of one hand, sharp but gentle blows are delivered between the shoulder blades. Foreign bodies such as pieces of small toys should be expelled, thus clearing the airway. Respirations may begin spontaneously, if not, artificial ventilation must be initiated immediately.

Accurate placement of the rescuer's hands during external cardiac compression will reduce the incidence of complications. The liver lies higher within the thoracic cavity under the lower sternum and xiphoid process. The chest wall is more pliable. Together, there is a danger of lacerating the liver during C.P.R.

Legal Implications

At the present time, a great deal of attention is being focused on medical-legal issues by physicians and nurses. Malpractice insurance for health care providers is skyrocketing to astronomical figures. Moral and legal issues may be of some concern to the rescuer(s).

In 1974, the Emergency Cardiac Care Committee not only standardized the techniques of administering C.P.R., but it also developed certain guidelines describing people who should be resuscitated. Persons suffering from long-term debilitating illnesses are not prime candidates for resuscitation.

Illinois is one of the forty states that has a Good Samaritan statute. These laws ensure that laymen who provide basic life support cannot be held liable if the victim suffers permanent damage or does not survive.

The general public is not legally obligated to perform C.P.R. techniques. However, if C.P.R. is initiated, the rescuers involved are obligated to perform it to the best of their ability. They are responsible for the victim until medical help arrives at the scene. Artificial circulatory and ventilatory support must be continued until it is no longer required, is considered futile, or until the rescuers' own health is endangered.

Conclusion

Coronary artery disease causes more than one-third of all deaths in the United States. Observation immediately after the onset of the coronary attack has proved pertinent to the understanding of the mechanism of sudden death. Early observation has also indicated the possibility of limiting the size of the damaged area of the heart and thus diminishing the incidence of complications. C.P.R. is a simple, lifesaving first aid technique that has been used to save thousands of victims who have had heart stoppage from heart conditions, electric shock, drowning, or even automobile accidents. Thousands of people are alive today who have suffered clinical death, but not biological death, because of swift initiation of C.P.R. The chances of survival for any victim will be increased as the percent of the total population adequately trained in these life support techniques is increased.

Thorough and careful training of the rescuers for successful applications of cardio-pulmonary resuscitation requires such teaching aids as written instructions, lectures, films, and demonstrations of artificial ventilation and external cardiac compression on life-size mannequins. Of utmost importance, though, is actual participation by the audience learners. Although not acrobatic in nature, placement of the rescuer's hands and maintaining proper body alignment is awkward at first to the inexperienced person, yet essential for C.P.R. to be administered properly and effectively. Several practice sessions need to be offered to allow participants to familiarize themselves with proper hand placement and timing. These rescue techniques cannot be learned and successfully applied without practice.

Cardio-pulmonary resuscitation can best be learned by formal enrollment in a first aid course offered in your community. Proper techniques are more readily learned with the use of life-size mannequins that are employed as teaching aids in most of these courses. For further information, call the local Red Cross or Y.M.C.A. For convenience, a list has been included towards the end of the book of the American Heart Association chapters across the country. Each chapter offers formal C.P.R. instruction. This book is merely an introduction to the terminology and techniques employed during C.P.R.——and is not to be used as a tool for certification.

Appendix I:
American Heart Association
Addresses

ALABAMA
P.O. Box 31085
Birmingham, Alabama 35222
205/324-2451

ALASKA
211 E. 4th Avenue
Anchorage, Alaska 99501
907/279-9541

ARIZONA
1445 E. Thomas
Phoenix, Arizona 85014
602/277-4846

ARKANSAS
909 W. 2nd Street
Little Rock, Arkansas 72201
501/375-9148

CALIFORNIA
805 Burlway Road
Burlingame, California 94010
415/342-5522

2405 West 8th Street
Los Angeles, California 90057
213/385-4231

COLORADO
4521 E. Virginia Avenue
Denver, Colorado 80222
303/399-2131

CONNECTICUT
71 Parker Avenue
Meriden, Connecticut 06450
203/634-4532

DELAWARE
1601 Concord Pike
Wilmington, Delaware 19803
302/654-5269

DISTRICT OF COLUMBIA
2233 Wisconsin Avenue
Washington, D.C. 20001
202/337-6400

FLORIDA
2828 Central Avenue
St. Petersburg, Florida 33712
813/894-6865

GEORGIA
2581 Piedmont Road, N.E.
Atlanta, Georgia 30324
404/261-2260

HAWAII
245 North Kukui Street
Honolulu, Hawaii 96817
808/538-7021

IDAHO
1301 South Capitol Blvd.
Boise, Idaho 83706
208/342-5621

ILLINOIS
1181 North Dirksen Parkway
Springfield, Illinois 62708
217/525-1350

20 North Wacker Drive
Chicago, Illinois 60606
312/346-4675
(covers DuPage,
Lake and Cook Counties)

INDIANA
222 South Downey Suite 222
Indianapolis, Indiana 46219
317/357-8622

IOWA
3810 Ingersoll Avenue
Des Moines, Iowa 50312
515/277-6371

KANSAS
5229 West 7th Street
Topeka, Kansas 66606
913/272-7056

KENTUCKY
333 Guthrie Street
Louisville, Kentucky 40202
502/587-8641

LOUISIANA
P.O. Box 19122
New Orleans, Louisiana 70179
504/827-1644

MAINE
20 Winter Street
Augusta, Maine 04330
207/623-8432

MARYLAND
10 South Street
Baltimore, Maryland 21202
301/539-0818

MASSACHUSETTS
33 Broad Street
Boston, Massachusetts 02109
617/227-2805

MICHIGAN
16310 West Twelve Mile Road
Southfield, Michigan 48076
313/557-9500

MINNESOTA
4701 West 77th Street
Minneapolis, Minnesota 55435
612/835-3300

MISSISSIPPI
P.O. Box 16063
(4830 E. McWillie Circle)
Jackson, Mississippi 39206
601/981-4721

MISSOURI
P.O. Box Q
601 East Broadway
Columbia, Missouri 65201
314/442-3193

MONTANA
510 1st Avenue North
Great Falls, Montana 59401
406/452-2362

NEBRASKA
3624 Farnam
Omaha, Nebraska 68131
402/346-0771

NEVADA
P.O. Box 1218
Chico, California 95926
916/342-4247

NEW HAMPSHIRE
54 South State Street
Concord, New Hampshire 03301
603/224-7461

NEW JERSEY
1525 Morris Avenue
Union, New Jersey 07083
201/688-4540

NEW MEXICO
142 Truman Street, N.E.
Albuquerque, New Mexico 87108
505/256-7335

NEW YORK (STATE)
3 West 29th Street
New York, New York 10001
212/686-3860

NEW YORK CITY
2 East 64th Street
New York, New York 10021
212/838-8800

NORTH CAROLINA
One Heart Circle
Chapel Hill, North Carolina 27514
919/968-4453

NORTH DAKOTA
1005 Twelfth Avenue, S.E.
Jamestown, North Dakota 58401
701/252-5122

NORTHEAST OHIO
1689 East 115th Street
Cleveland, Ohio 44106
216/791-7500

OHIO
10 East Town Street
Columbus, Ohio 43215
614/224-4276-77

OKLAHOMA
800 Northeast 15th Street
Oklahoma City, Oklahoma 73111
405/236-5534

OREGON
1500 S.W. 12th Avenue
Portland, Oregon 97201
503/226-2575

PENNSYLVANIA
2743 North Front Street
Harrisburg, Pennsylvania 17110
717/238-0895

PUERTO RICO
554 Cabo Alverio Street
San Juan, Puerto Rico 00919
809/763-8102
809/763-8275

RHODE ISLAND
40 Broad Street
Pawtucket, Rhode Island 02860
401/728-5300

SOUTH CAROLINA
2864 Devine Street
Columbia, South Carolina 29205
803/771-4820

TENNESSEE
1720 Westend Building
Nashville, Tennessee 37203
615/320-0390

TEXAS
860 North Highway 183
Austin, Texas 78757
512/836-7220

UTAH
250 E. 1st Street South
Salt Lake City, Utah 84111
801/322-5601

VERMONT
56 Church Street
Rutland, Vermont 05701
802/773-9300

VIRGINIA
316 E. Clay Street
Richmond, Virginia 23219
804/643-7391

WASHINGTON
333 First Avenue West
Seattle, Washington 98119
206/285-2415

WEST VIRGINIA
211 35th Street, S.E.
Charleston, West Virginia 25304
304/346-5381

WISCONSIN
795 North Van Buren Street
Milwaukee, Wisconsin 53202
414/271-9999

WYOMING
217 W. 18th Street
Cheyenne, Wyoming 82001
307/632-1746

Appendix II:
Glossary of Medical Terms

ABDOMEN - the part of the body below the rib cage containing the liver, spleen and intestines

ACUTE - sudden onset

AFFERENT - nerve impulses traveling towards the brain

AIRWAY - nose or mouth carrying air to the lungs

ALVEOLUS - sac-like structure where oxygen and carbon dioxide are exchanged in the lungs

ANATOMY - structure of the human body

ANGINA - chest pain or pressure

ANOXIA - insufficient oxygen

ANTERIOR - front

ANTERIOR-POSTERIOR - front to back

ANTI - against

AORTA - the largest artery in the body carrying blood to the organs and cells

APEX - pointed portion of the heart

ARREST - cessation or stoppage

ARRYTHMIA - irregular heartbeat

ARTERIOLE - smaller branch of an artery

ARTERIOSCLEROSIS - loss of elasticity and hardening of the arterial walls

ARTERY - vessel carrying blood from the heart to the body tissues

ASPHYXIA - death caused by ineffective exchange of oxygen and carbon dioxide in the lungs

ASPIRATE - inhale secretions into the lungs

ASTHMA - difficulty breathing characterized by wheezing due to bronchospasm

ATHEROMA - plaque deposits in the arterial wall

ATHEROSCLEROSIS - formation and collection of deposits containing cholesterol and fatty acids in the arterial wall

ATRIA - plural of the atrium

ATRIUM - top chamber of the heart collecting blood from the body and lungs

ATTACK - sudden onset of symptoms or illness

A.V. NODE - special nerve fibers controlling impulses delivered to the ventricles

BLOOD - fluid transporting oxygen to the tissues from the heart

BLOOD PRESSURE - pressure along the elastic walls of the arteries

BRACHIAL - large artery in the arm located at the bend of the elbow used to measure the blood pressure

BRADY - slow; pertaining to the heart-bradycardia, abnormal slowness of the heart rate and pulse

BRONCHI - plural of bronchus

BRONCHIOLE - smaller segment of the bronchus

BRONCHOSPIROMETER - instrument used to determine the functional capacity of the lungs

BRONCHUS - one of the large tubes carrying air into and out of the lungs

CAPILLARY - microscopic cells where arterioles and venules join and carbon dioxide and oxygen exchange takes place

CARDIO - pertaining to the heart

CARDIO-VASCULAR - the heart and blood vessels composing the circulatory system

CAROTID - the large artery supplying blood to the head located in the neck approximately one and one-half inches to either side of the Adam's apple.

c.c. - cubic centimeter - measurement used to determine the volume of circulating blood

CEPHALO - head

CILIA - thin hairs found lining the mucous membrances of the nose

CIRCULATION - movement in a circle such as the blood

COLLATERAL - compensatory mechanism of the heart whereby smaller branches of end-arteries forming interconnected pathways are established as a result of an occlusion

COMPLICATION - symptoms or a disease resulting from a previous condition

COMPRESSION - pressing together

CONDUCTION - transmission of nerve impulses along a pathway

CONSTRICTION - narrowing of a blood vessel

CONTRACTION - shortening of the muscle fibers causing movement

CORONARY - relating to the heart; crown-arteries surrounding the heart delivering blood directly to it for its own supply

CYANOTIC - bluish color due to insufficient oxygen

DEATH - cessation of life; clinical - the absence of vital signs such as pulse and respirations; biological - irreversible changes at the cellular level resulting in absolute death

DIAPHORESIS - profuse sweating

DIAPHRAGM - dome shaped muscle separating the thoracic cage and its contents from the abdominal organs

DIASTOLE - the relaxing stage of the cardiac cycle where the chambers fill; pressure—normal resting pressure constantly present along the walls of the arteries

DYSPNEA - difficulty breathing

EFFERENT - progressing away from a reference point such as the brain

ELECTROCARDIOGRAM - recording of the heart's electrical activity

END-ARTERY - an artery that does not join with another, i.e. coronary artery

ENDOCARDIUM - innermost lining of the heart

EPICARDIUM - outermost lining of the heart

ESOPHAGUS - tube extending from the pharynx to the stomach

GASTRO-INTESTINAL - pertaining to the stomach and intestines

HEALTH - a state of physical, mental and social well-being

HEART - the muscular organ of the cardio-vascular system that maintains the body's circulation

HEMOGLOBIN - the oxygen-carrying pigment of the blood

HEREDITY - the transmission of certain traits from parent to offspring

HORMONE - a chemical substance produced by the body which has a specific effect on an organ, i.e. cholesterol

HYPERTENSION - elevated blood pressure

HYPOXIA - abnormally low concentration of oxygen

INFARCT - localized area of ischemic necrosis produced by occlusion of the arterial blood supply; i.e. myocardial infarction—formation of an infarct in the heart muscle due to interruption of the blood supply to the area

INFERIOR - lower; such as the lower segment of the lungs

INFERIOR VENA CAVA - large vein transporting blood from the lower portion of the body returning it to the heart

ISCHEMIA - deficiency of blood due to constriction or obstruction of a blood vessel

LARYNX - air passageway between the pharynx and trachea containing the vocal cords

LATERAL - pertaining to the side

LOBE - specific portion of an organ such as the lung

LUNG - spongy organ where oxygen and carbon dioxide are exchanged

MASSAGE - compressing the heart between the sternum and spinal column during C.P.R.

MEDULLA - respiratory control center in the brain

MESOMORPH - person of short stature with large, thick bones

METABOLISM - process whereby the body cells use oxygen to produce energy and carbon dioxide is released

MYOCARDIUM - thick middle layer of the heart muscle responsible for its pumping action

NERVE - specialized tissue cells capable of transmitting impulses, conveying sensation and originating movement

OCCLUSION - complete blockage of blood flow

PALPITATION - fluttering sensation of the heart

PERICARDIAL SAC - protective fluid-filled sac encompassing the heart

PHARYNX - cylindrical tube joining the back of the nose and mouth to form the throat

PULMONARY - relating to the lungs or respiratory system

PULSE - rhythmical tapping sensation felt over an artery indicating the heartbeat

RESPIRATION - the movement of air into and out of the lungs; the exchange of oxygen and carbon dioxide across the alveolar-capillary membrane

RESUSCITATION - restoration of life

RHYTHM - regularity of occurrence

S.A. NODE - pacemaker of the heart controlling the rate and rhythm of the heartbeat

SCLEROSIS - hardening of the arteries

SEDENTARY - lack of regular daily exercise

SIGN - an indication exhibited by one person and objectively perceived by another

SPASM - intermittent constriction of an artery usually resulting from physical activity or stress

STERNUM - breastbone located in the upper middle part of the chest

SUPERIOR - upper; such as the upper lobe of the lungs

SUPERIOR VENA CAVA - large vein transporting blood from the head and upper part of the body returning it to the heart

SYMPTOM - subjective feeling only experienced by that individual

SYNDROME - a disease process characterized by a combination of symptoms

SYNERGISTIC - the combined effects of two agents working together

SYSTOLE - the contracting stage of the cardiac cycle where the chambers force the blood out into the circulation; pressure—measurement of pressure along the arterial walls as the heart contracts

TACHY - fast; pertaining to the heart-tachycardia, abnormally fast heartbeat and pulse

THORAX - upper portion of the body between the neck and diaphragm containing the lungs and heart

THROMBOSIS - solid mass such as a blood clot obstructing blood flow

TRACHEA - that portion of the cylindrical tube known as the windpipe

VEIN - blood vessel transporting blood from the body tissues back to the heart

VENTILATION - exchange of oxygen and carbon dioxide

VENTRICLE - lower chamber of the heart forcing the blood to the lungs and the body tissues

XIPHOID - thin sword-shaped piece of bone forming the lower part of the sternum

Appendix III:
A Condensed Recap

IS THERE CARDIAC ARREST?

What To Look For

1. STATE OF COLLAPSE OR UNCONSCIOUSNESS

2. PULSE

Check carotid, brachial, or radial artery for pulse. Carotid (neck) is easiest to locate.

3. BREATHING

Has victim stopped breathing? Check for rise and fall of chest. Place ear next to nose to feel breath.

4. PUPILS

Pupils will be dilated (larger) and will not respond to light.

5. SKIN COLOR

Skin will have bluish tint due to lack of oxygen in the blood.

**CARDIAC ARREST SHOULD BE
CONSIDERED WHENEVER A PERSON
SUDDENLY COLLAPSES OR LOSES
CONSCIOUSNESS**

CARDIAC ARREST ADULT

What To Do

1. AMBULANCE

Call or have someone else call an ambulance. Be sure to tell them you have a cardiac arrest victim.

2. LAY VICTIM ON FLOOR

Victim should be on his back on a firm foundation.

3. CLEAR AIRWAY

Make sure there is no obstruction in the airway. Tilt head back and make sure tongue is not blocking airway.

ONE RESCUER

4. 4 QUICK VENTILATIONS

5. BEGIN C.P.R. CYCLE

15 compressions
2 ventilations
15 compressions
2 ventilations . . .

6. MAINTAIN C.P.R. CYCLE

TWO RESCUERS

4. 2 QUICK VENTILATIONS

5. BEGIN C.P.R. CYCLE

5 compressions
1 ventilation
5 compressions
1 ventilation . . .

6. MAINTAIN C.P.R. CYCLE

CARDIAC ARREST CHILD

What To Do

1. AMBULANCE

Call or have someone else call an ambulance. Be sure to tell them you have a child or infant cardiac arrest victim.

2. LAY VICTIM ON FLOOR OR TABLE

Be sure back is supported by a pillow or the rescuer's hand.

3. CLEAR AIRWAY

Make sure there is no obstruction in the airway. Tilt head back BUT less extremely than for an adult. Make sure tongue is not blocking airway.

4. 2 QUICK VENTILATIONS

5. BEGIN C.P.R. CYCLE

5 compressions
1 ventilation
5 compressions
1 ventilation

COMPRESSIONS:
80–100 per minute
Higher on chest than for adult
Heel of one hand for child
Use index and middle fingers for infant

VENTILATIONS:
20 per minute, 1 every 3 seconds
Rescuer's mouth covers victim's nose and mouth completely
Deliver small ventilations

6. MAINTAIN C.P.R. CYCLE

Index